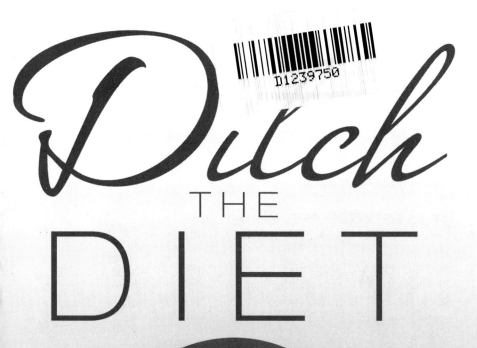

Ditch

THE

DIET

HOW YOUR
FRUSTRATION
CAN LEAD TO
**FREEDOM AND
PERMANENT
WEIGHT LOSS**

LEAH CAMPIÁN

POWERED BY

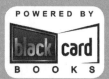

black card
B O O K S

Author: Leah Campián
Title: Ditch the Diet
ISBN: 978-1-77204-019-7
Category: HEALTH & FITNESS/Diet & Nutrition/Weight Loss

Publisher: Black Card Books
Division of Gerry Robert Enterprises Inc.
Suite 214, 5-18 Ringwood Drive
Stouffville, Ontario, Canada, L4A 0N2
International Calling: +1 877 280 8536
www.blackcardbooks.com

....

Ditch
THE
DIET

HOW YOUR FRUSTRATION CAN LEAD TO
FREEDOM AND PERMANENT WEIGHT LOSS

LEAH CAMPIÁN

POWERED BY

B O O K S

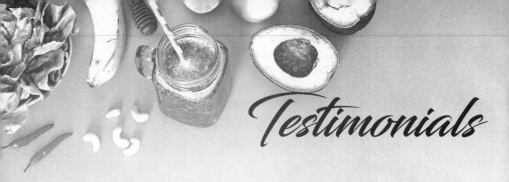

Testimonials

"When you have tried everything and it has not worked out the way you wanted, forgive yourself for being human! With this simple and effective approach, Leah Campián has finally got the solution to the 'mental side' of releasing your weight and staying healthy for life. As someone who has lost almost 100 pounds FIVE times in my life, only to gain MORE back each time, I can attest to the mental strength needed to keep it off, this SIXTH time, FOREVER! Your desire for health, your will to do it, and the ultimate picture you have for your health will be realized by following this powerful, practical, and proven advice on getting and staying healthy."

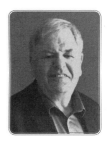

—Barry Spilchuk
Co-author of *A Cup of Chicken Soup for the Soul*
Founder of www.TheLEGACY.club

"This book is a great read! It is thoughtful and insightful, yet practical and easy to follow. I like how Leah makes connections and paints the bigger picture of what could be and how to get there. Being an expert in the wellness industry, I believe this is a great book to add to your collection!"

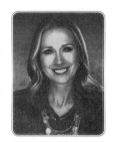

—Gina Van Luven
Bestselling Author and Board Certified Health Coach
www.ginavanluven.com

"With her book *Ditch the Diet*, Culinary Nutrition Expert Leah Campián has simplified how to achieve the objective of optimal health. Outlining how and why diets continue to fail, Leah offers an evidence-based and approachable strategy to achieve health goals. Her complete lifestyle plan will inspire readers to see that health is within reach. I share in the philosophy that Leah champions—that there is no one way of eating and living for all of us. This book empowers readers to ditch the diet forever and start living a healthful, inspired life."

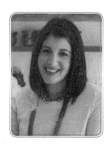

—Meghan Telpner
Bestselling Author of *The UnDiet Cookbook*
Founder of The Academy of Culinary Nutrition
www.meghantelpner.com

"I had the fortune of hearing about Coach Leah's book during a phase where I had almost totally gotten away from mindful eating. Life quickly gets busy, and it's so easy for me to slip back into bad habits.

While reading her book, I was hooked from the first page, seeing how she combined her creativity, passion, and expert knowledge into such an easy read. Therefore, if you're looking for quick, yet practical solutions for staying healthy and living a better life, go ahead and ditch the diet using this amazing guide that delivers a winning one-two punch... with so much less pain!"

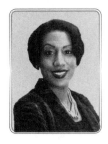

—C-A Washington
Executive Director of Image & Etiquette Institute
Author of *The Art of A.R.C. – Appearance, Relationships & Credibility: Shaping Your Image for the Next Level*
www.imageandetiquetteinstitute.com

"In *Ditch the Diet*, Leah shows the reader how taking ownership of their health is the best investment they could ever make in themselves. She shares how to overcome excuses and mental blocks, identify the real causes of weight gain, and how to discover what you're REALLY hungry for so you can keep the weight off for good!"

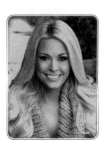

—Cynthia Pasquella-Garcia
Founder and Director of the Institute of Transformational Nutrition
www.cynthiapasquella.com

Foreword

On occasion, a new discovery in human health creates a paradigm shift, a change in the way we think about the topic. This is called translational research. And the scientists tell us that the average, not the exception, but the average length of time from when translational research is published before the Doctor down the street is using this way of thinking, this new technology, to help patients is 17 years. 17 years![1] The time between the first time someone said, "Cholesterol may have something to do with heart disease," or a researcher discovered that "trans fats cause more inflammation in the body," or that "smoking was bad for you," or that "wheat creates problems in the gut for every human," or when the first papers clearly demonstrated the facts and the time we as humans began using this information in our quest to get healthier is 17 years.

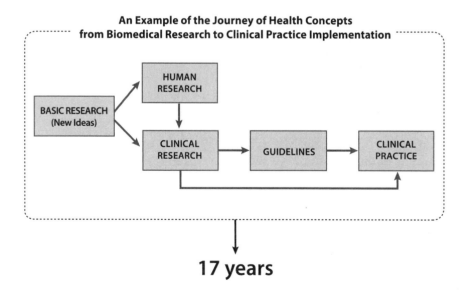

An Example of the Journey of Health Concepts from Biomedical Research to Clinical Practice Implementation

HUMAN RESEARCH

BASIC RESEARCH (New Ideas)

CLINICAL RESEARCH

GUIDELINES

CLINICAL PRACTICE

17 years

---

1   Z. S. Morris, S. Wooding, J. Grant, "The Answer Is 17 years, What Is the Question: Understanding Time Lags in Translational Research," J R Soc Med 104, 12 (Dec 2011): 510–20.

And now the results of this "head in the sand" resistance that we have had as people are threatening our survival. Here are two studies that put this into perspective. The World Wildlife Fund[2] recently published that between 1970 and 2012, in 42 years, there has been on average a 58 percent reduction in numbers of all vertebrate species on the planet. Fifty-eight percent of everything with a spine (birds, insects, fish, mammals, etc.) is gone. Gone in the last 42 years. For terrestrials (things that fly), the loss is 38 percent. For those near fresh water, it's 75 percent. Of every vertebrate species living near fresh water, 75 percent of them have disappeared in the last 42 years. Gone. Why so high a number? They're drinking the water. And if you were drinking the water coming out of the streams or rivers by your home, you'd get cancer quicker. And you'd be unable to reproduce, just like the animals.

That's pretty frightening, but as is true with most numbers, only a few understand what numbers mean. For most of us, if it's not causing a problem right now, we tend to **forget about it.**

And here's the next statistic that puts this into perspective and takes it out of the theoretical and right down to what's got you by the cojones right now. In a study looking at many earlier studies on one theme or topic, a meta-analysis of 180+ studies on the topic of sperm count in healthy men—and mind you these are healthy men, not infertile men—between 1973 and 2011, there has been a 59 percent reduction in sperm count in men. Across the board. 59 percent. Scientists tell us they start worrying about the extinction of a species at 72 percent. And we're at 59% loss in 38 years.[3]

---

2   Living Planet Index, http://www.livingplanetindex.org/home/index (accessed January 26, 2018).

3   H. Levine, N. Jørgensen, A. Martino-Andrade, J. Mendiola, D. Weksler-Derri, I. Mindlis, R. Pinotti, S. H. Swan, "Temporal Trends in Sperm Count: A Systematic Review and Meta-Regression Analysis," *Hum Reprod Update* 1; 23, 6 (Nov 2017): 646–659.

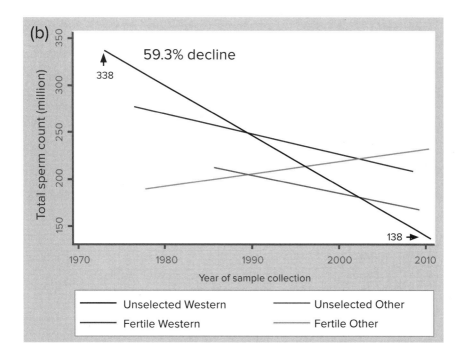

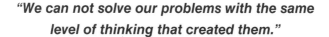

What's needed is a paradigm shift for the general public. We have to think outside the box of the preconceived notions we may have. This quote is attributed to Einstein (he was a pretty smart guy and worth listening to). His quote:

"We can not solve our problems with the same level of thinking that created them."

As a people, we have to up our game in terms of how we think about food, the environment, chemicals we're exposed to... and all the evidence suggests that is not likely to happen. That we're all locked in to how we think. We're sure our line of thinking is right and most everyone else is wrong. Well, the result of that type of thinking has gotten us into the mess we're in today.

This is very important because it is the only way that I can think of to initiate change at a global level. To literally save the planet for our children and grandchildren.

We all know some or most of the things that are good for us and what is not—why don't we act more often on what is good for us? I've said this many times over the years: "Humans are the only species on the planet who find something that's good for us, and we stop doing it." That question is a book in itself. What's important right now is this: What can we do to change our paradigm and the way I and my family think about food so that it's effective and we all get healthier?

What I like so much about Leah Campián's book *Ditch the Diet* is that her message is saturated with "change your paradigm" information. One of the studies she refers to is an excellent example of how when we change how we think about a topic, it changes how we act. Two groups of college students were taught about food and health. The group that learned about all the dangers of poor choices continued eating poorly and even got a little worse. The information had very little effect on making change. The college group taught about the impact of food choices on environmental, ethical, social justice, cultural, political and agricultural issues, and had discussion groups on these topics actually changed their food choices, began eating more vegetables, less meat, less fast foods and reported being healthier.[4]

We have to think differently in order to be successful at acting differently.

---

4   E. B. Hekler, C. D. Garnder, and T. N. Robinson, "Effects of a College Course About Food and Society on Students' Eating Behaviors," *American Journal of Preventative Medicine,* 38, no. 5 (May 2010): 543–47.

- Discussions around the family table at dinner about tonight's dinner, for example. What's the root vegetable tonight? We all should have at least one root vegetable per day in our diet,
- Did everyone get some fermented vegetables today? If not, here's some on the table. Everyone should have at least 1 tablespoon of fermented vegetables per day (sauerkraut, kimchi, miso, etc.).
- How hard was it for Dad today in his business lunch meeting to find something healthy on the menu and what was the thought process he went through to make his selection?
- Engaging with like-minded people on Facebook group chats who are learning new things all the time.

Ditch the Diet is full of these little pearls that will empower, encourage, and guide the reader into making healthier choices because you want to, not because you have to.

This book brings a treasure trove of guidance in developing a new mindset and will make a valuable contribution to your health library.

Towards better health for all,

Tom O' Bryan

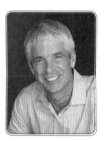

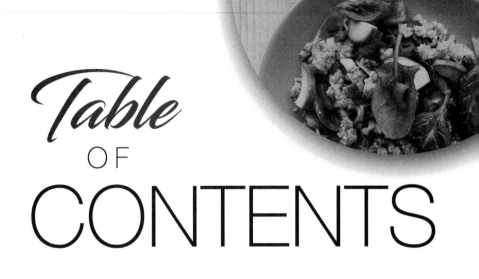

Table
OF
CONTENTS

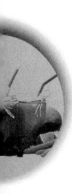

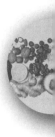

Part 2: Nourishing Your Spirit, Soul, and Mind

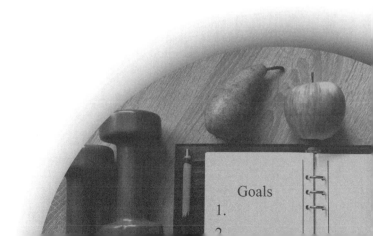

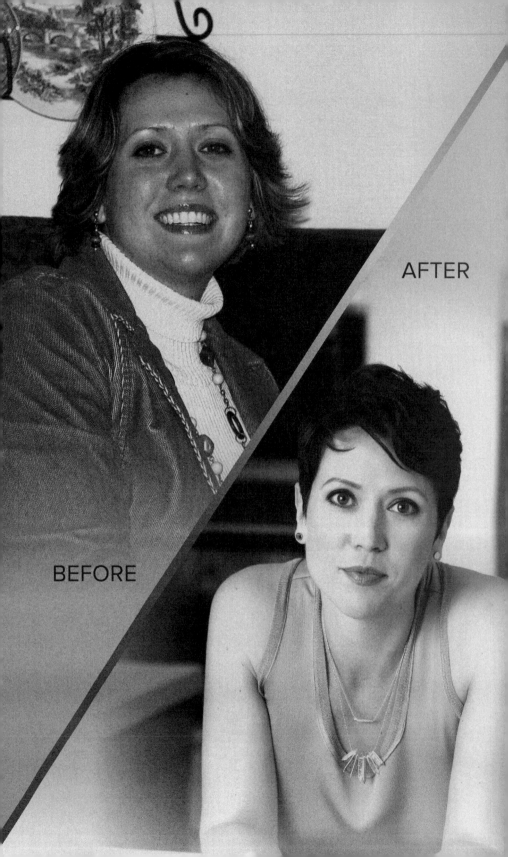

AFTER

BEFORE

Preface

Are you tired of jumping from one diet to the next only to find yourself more frustrated, exhausted, confused, and worse than before? Maybe you've found diets that work but only if you stick to their strict rules, disappointed to see your weight yo-yoing as you dip in and out of die-hard discipline. Or maybe you never bothered with diets in the first place but now you're ready for some permanent change. Whatever your reason for picking up this book, I'm glad you did, and I'm excited to share with you how to gain permanent freedom and transformation!

Like many of you, I've tried a lot of diets, stuck to them unwaveringly, went through the mundane scripts faithfully, suffered while watching others enjoy life, jealous of the skinny girl who could eat anything, saw some temporary results, learned some things along the way, and finally learned that I was better off without them after all! Not to mention that I had no idea that my health problems were directly related to my diet and lifestyle. Today, I am one of the most fortunate people I know! I get to use my passion to help others transform their lives, but it wasn't always this way.

As a child, I can remember being called "Fatty Bread" and "the heavier twin." I wasn't really fat, but having another one of me who was thinner made me the "chubby" one. Following in the steps of a teenager I looked up to as my role model, I started dieting at age 12 and continued until my early 30s. I tried many diets, saw many ups and downs, and was never satisfied with my body, even when I was at my lowest weight. As much as I obsessed, I just couldn't figure out how to maintain the weight loss. I thought that seeing skinny models in magazines would keep me motivated to make healthy choices and improve self-control.

I was intrigued by nutritional information, and the more I tried to understand it all, the more confused I became with the contradicting nutritional information I learned. "Who is right?" "How do I know who to believe?" "Which diet will work for me?" In adulthood, I struggled to maintain not only my weight but my energy levels and overall health as well. I've battled chronic fatigue, afternoon slumps, the munchies, body aches and pains, and sports injuries. I've suffered from insomnia, acne, acid reflux, chronic infections, colds, and migraines. Doctors' visits were almost monthly, for one issue or another, with symptoms that would either come back later or that I could never shake off no matter how much medicine they gave me. Every day I was taking an antihistamine, a nasal spray steroid, steroid eye drops, with occasional to frequent use of anti-acids, migraine medication, antibiotics for various types of infections, and acne treatments. I realized something wasn't right when one of my employees said, "Leah, for someone who eats so 'healthy' and works out all the time, you sure do go to the doctor a lot!" And you know what? She was right! That's when I finally decided to find the answers myself. That's when I knew I was ready for a true transformation—a *lasting* one.

My transformation certainly didn't happen overnight. It took many years of studying, listening, learning, and research. While studying to become a Certified Transformational Nutrition Coach and Certified Culinary Nutrition Expert, my eyes were opened to new alternatives to health care. It blew my mind to learn about things like "epigenetics," the idea that we can "turn on" and "turn off" certain genes with changes in diet and lifestyle. Many of the health problems I was experiencing I chalked up to my mother passing them along to me, since she had the same issues. I felt like I was doomed to that fate no matter what I did, that I'd only be able to manage the symptoms but never really get rid of the diseases and wholly get better. Yet as I was empowered to practice what I learned from holistic health studies, I felt better, I looked better, and my life and that of my family's changed forever. I can happily say that I generally don't get sick anymore, take no medications, and stay energized throughout the day. I've learned to listen to my body and give it what it needs to thrive and be vibrant. When I do start to feel bad, I take note, make the necessary adjustments in my lifestyle or food intake, and the sickness never evolves into anything more than a sign from my body that it needs care or that I need to slow down. I want you to know the same is possible for you too. You can have the body and the life you've dreamed of. It's not as complicated as you may think.

> We will all go astray, but the difference in our results is what we do when we fail. Do you fail forward, using the experience as an opportunity to teach you, or do you use it as an excuse to take another step back?

I truly practice what I preach, not for fear of being an impostor, but for fear of going backward, of not feeling well, not looking my best, not being my best so I can serve my purpose in this world. Am I perfect? By no means. Do I fail? Absolutely! We will all go astray, but the difference in our results is what we do when we fail. Do you fail forward, using the experience as an opportunity to teach you, or do you use it as an excuse to take another step back? That's why it's so important to understand all that you are—mind, body, spirit (soul)—for without this understanding, life is like a journey without a map… very confusing and difficult to see where you might end up. That kind of journey leaves you with no choice. On the other hand, when you have the knowledge, understanding, and tools you need for the journey, you have choices. You can create the life you were meant to live, find fulfillment in everything you do, and be the person the world is waiting to see. Every day is a choice to live anew, vibrantly and passionately! If you're ready for that journey, keep reading. This book's for you!

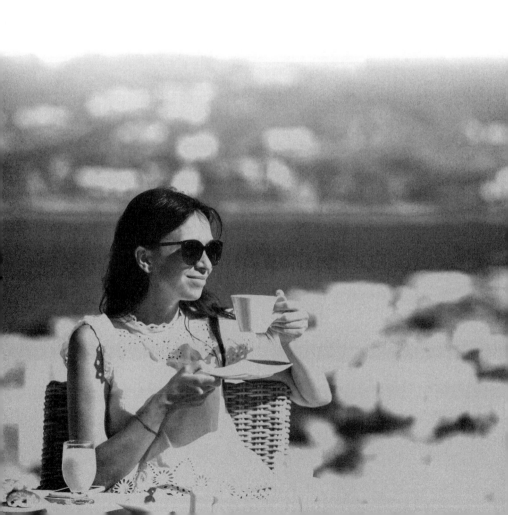

Introduction

WHY YOU SHOULD DITCH THE DIET

Ever wonder why you just can't stick to your diet? Do you feel like you're just jumping from one diet to the next with no lasting results? Well, my friend, you're certainly not alone! Your frustration is felt by many others struggling to lose weight, increase their energy, and improve their health. The following pages will address whether diets are really the right approach to managing your weight, whether they are good for you, and why so few of us are able to stick with what's good for us.

In reality, the issue is the diet, not you. Diets don't work because:

❖ they don't promote authenticity within us;

❖ they create obsessive behaviors like counting, controlling, denying, resenting, regretting, and negative thoughts;

❖ they lower our self-esteem when we try and fail;

❖ they encourage a cycle of disconnect between the mind and the body, causing us not to hear the voice within, creating a greater gap between who we are and who we want to be, abandoning our own intuitions rather than developing them;

❖ they don't encourage us to get in touch with our feelings and emotions so we can listen to our bodies and do what is best for ourselves in that moment;

- they don't create awareness and mindfulness, as we learn to become robots, with each step a controlled and calculated order to follow;

- they tell us that there are "good" and "bad" foods, that we are good or bad for the food choices we make, that we are not good enough, thin enough, beautiful enough;

- they promote body image issues, as they cause us to feel that we need them to "fix" ourselves in order to look a certain way;

- they don't encourage us to accept and embrace the natural phases of life where the body changes;

- they encourage a bad relationship with food—their restrictive nature can create cycles of binge eating, fatigue, headaches, depression, anxiety, hormonal imbalances, and joint pain to autoimmune reactions like allergies, irritable bowel syndrome, colitis, diabetes, and heart disease;

- they set unrealistic expectations for everyone—not all diets work the same way for everyone;

- they don't encourage self-compassion and self-love; in fact, they often encourage self-hate;

- they don't encourage us to understand our individually unique dietary and nutritional needs;

- they create significant stress, which causes further dietary issues and even disease.

A DIET	DITCHING THE DIET
❖ Tends to address the symptoms	❖ Addresses the *root cause*
❖ Focuses only on the body and food	❖ Has a 3D focus on the *mind, body, spirit*
❖ Has a one-size-fits-all approach	❖ Is a *unique* approach for the individual
❖ Is restricting and depriving	❖ Is about enhancing benefits for *thriving*
❖ Causes negative feelings	❖ Causes *positive* feelings
❖ Focuses on what you're giving up	❖ Focuses on what you're *gaining*
❖ Promotes self-hate	❖ Promotes *self-love*
❖ Is depleting	❖ Is giving
❖ Drains	❖ Energizes
❖ Is stressful	❖ Is enjoyable
❖ Might bring temporary satisfaction	❖ Is permanently rewarding

Ultimately, diets don't work! They don't allow us to know ourselves authentically, to accept ourselves for who we are, to love ourselves as we are, to be patient with ourselves as we grow, to cope with lifelong behavioral issues, to enjoy the different stages of our lives, to live in the present moment, and to relish all the feelings brought on by each experience in order to live life by being the fullest, most expressive versions of ourselves.

So far, I've focused on what doesn't work; however, my goal throughout the book is to compare what *doesn't* work with what *does* work. As you read through each chapter, you'll learn what worked for me and many others, and ways to explore what will work for you too. You'll see a lot of topics you may not have thought to be connected to one's health or even weight loss, but I will explain how they are not only connected but also essential for your success. Keep in mind, though, that I am sharing what has and hasn't worked for me and many others, but *not* for everyone, an important point we'll discuss in the next chapter. It's not my goal to try to save you; instead, I'm trying to *empower* you with the necessary awareness, mindset, and knowledge to set you up for success!

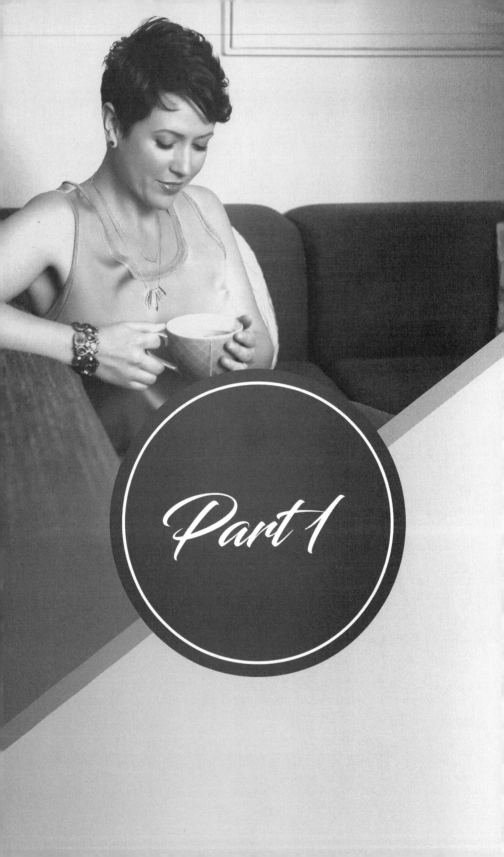

Part 1

Nourishing
YOUR
BODY
AND
MIND

This section of the book covers individual uniqueness, body image, values, food systems, making decisions, mind-body connection, mindful eating, movement, diet traps, mechanisms of weight loss, medication, food, and supplementation.

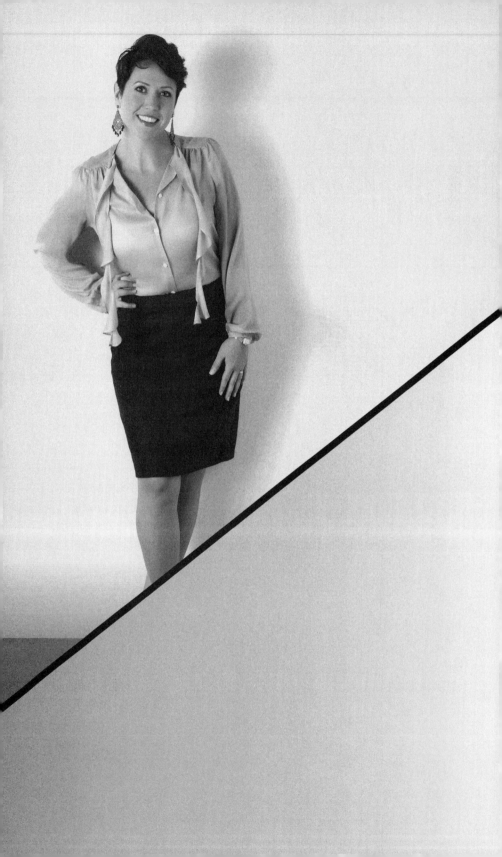

What Doesn't Work:
One-Size-Fits-All Approach

"To maintain your health, you have to want to be healthy because of your own pride and self-worth, then make a commitment to it. You have to consider the equation of food, sleep, stress, and exercise that's right for yourself to maintain your own health. It involves giving yourself permission to take steps to get there, even though it may take longer than expected."[5]

—Andy Levitt, CEO of Purple Carrot

You probably picked up this book with the hope that it wouldn't be another one-size-fits-all approach, and that you could finally obtain optimum health and permanent weight loss without following yet another diet! Or maybe you're on the other side of the fence: You just can't believe it's possible! Maybe you're feeling both. Whatever

---

5   Andy Levitt, interview with author on July 18, 2017.

your reason, I want to be sure we're on the same page in understanding the issue with dieting. By starting here together, we can all understand the rest of the book much better.

First, I believe that diets don't improve your life and health, but rather diminish them. Dieting is as destructive to your body as it is to your mind and spirit. The consequences of trying to implement short-term patches as solutions to long-term problems can be disastrous on many levels. Here are a few reasons why.

We Are All Unique Individuals

Our uniqueness makes us invaluable. Few of us truly understand and embrace the fact that God created us as unique individuals. On a recent trip to Morocco, my sister purchased a beautiful bracelet. When she gave it to me, she recounted her experience in negotiating the price, which started *very* high. The seller and maker of this prized possession declared, "It's hand-made! It's not like any other bracelet!" My sister, with her fine negotiating skills, replied, "Well, get a machine!" That story makes me laugh every time I look at the bracelet and think of its uniqueness and true value.

Many of us prefer to just fit in and look like everyone else. This need to belong is natural, but renouncing our uniqueness isn't the way to go about it. Instead, we should celebrate and honor our uniqueness by rejecting the industrial mass approach to everything, whether it is producing bracelets or shoes or delivering health care and education.

One of the major concerns with the one-size-fits-all approach in health care, nutrition, etc. is that the results will not be the same for everyone. This has very serious implications on many levels. Treatments are wrong and therefore inefficient; results that could be positive are negative; people who trust the health care system to take care of their health get confused and disheartened when they go through repeated treatment protocols and their health doesn't improve. When applying such a universal approach to weight control, for example, those who get negative results through no fault of their own feel as though they've failed, as though their personal worth is diminished. That's a very dangerous state of mind that further weakens a person's ability to make changes and focus on improving their condition. We're all unique, with different genetic responses, different motivators and interests, different reactions to the same stimuli, so our aim at health should be *centered on our uniqueness*.

Comparisons Can Be Dangerous

It is not unusual for people to share what worked for them, recommending that you follow their "recipe." That's not always a bad idea, as long as you understand your uniqueness. It's unsafe and counterproductive to assume the same method will work for you and to compare yourself to others. The comparison mindset can cause feelings of being either less than or better than someone else, rather than being centered on our own God-given uniqueness and on becoming the best version of ourselves. The feelings derived from comparisons can lead to two extremes—unhappiness or arrogance—neither of which will lead to healthy and happy lives.

I acknowledge that it's a constant internal struggle to look a certain way or even fit within certain measurements. I remember looking at magazines almost daily, feeling bad about myself because I didn't look like the skinny models whose photos are always edited and polished. I somehow thought that seeing them would motivate me to do what it takes to have a body like that. But I would never have a body like theirs—I'm short and muscular. It's just not possible (without Photoshop).

Now, however, I don't care what my BMI or weight is. I don't measure them. Comparisons and the wrong measurements take us further away

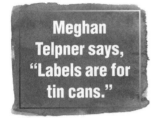

Meghan Telpner says, "Labels are for tin cans."

from knowing ourselves and being our authentic selves. We are not a number. We are so much more than our bodies. We are unique eternal creatures that God made with a unique purpose. Why would we want to be anything or anybody else?

We Have a Tendency to Oversimplify

We want to label everything and everyone. One of my teachers and the author of the book *UnDiet* and *The UnDiet Cookbook,* Meghan Telpner says, "Labels are for tin cans."[6] So why do we label each other? It makes us feel safe and in control when we can put everything in a box. The truth is, black and white is easier. It doesn't require as much thought and discernment as working in the gray. But that line of thinking keeps us trying to fit into something we're not, instead of taking the time to find what's a good fit for us individually. The food pyramid is such an example. This guideline originated from faulty science and government subsidies; in other words, the government wants us to eat what it's putting its money into, but it's not the government's job to tell us what and how much to eat, and that guideline is definitely not right for everyone. (For information on how the food pyramid came to be, read *Death by Food Pyramid* by Denise Minger.[7])

---

6   Meghan Telpner, *UnDiet: The Shiny, Happy, Vibrant, Gluten-Free, Plant-Based Way to Look Better, Feel Better, and Live Better Each and Every Day!* (Guilford: Skirt!, 2013), 62–63.

7   Denise Minger, *Death by Food Pyramid: How Shoddy Science, Sketchy Politics and Shady Special Interests Ruined Your Health...and How to Reclaim It!* (Malibu: Primal Blueprint Publishing, 2013).

There Is No Cookie-Cutter Solution

Cookie-cutter solutions are easy, efficient, and cheap. Customization has a cost, and unfortunately we go with what we think we can afford. Think about buying a house. We all want ours to be different from everyone else's, but we're settling for a choice of only three to five different models because that's what we can afford. When it comes to your health, the cookie-cutter solution just won't cut it (pun intended). You deserve better than that. So I invite you to stop trying to fit into a mold that has been made for the masses. Instead, you can learn to listen to your body, satisfying both your wants and needs. This will be covered in more detail in another chapter.

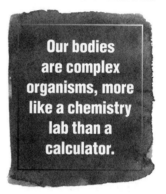

Our bodies are complex organisms, more like a chemistry lab than a calculator.

It's More Than Just Simple Math

Another confusing part of this trend is the belief that our bodies work like a simple math problem. We've all heard that weight loss boils down to calories in and calories out, but our bodies are complex organisms, more like a chemistry lab than a calculator. So you can stop counting all those calories now! Again, this is just another form of measurement, pushing you further away from knowing yourself, listening to your body in every moment, and honoring what it is telling you. Rest assured, there's a better way to lose weight than continuously counting calories, and I'm going to show you how.

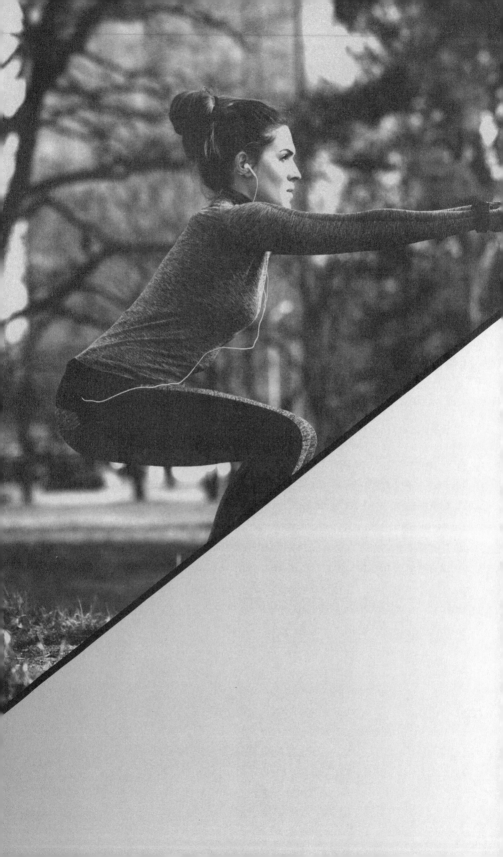

What Doesn't Work:
Depending on Willpower Alone

"Two hard truths:
1. People are 'creatures of habit.'
2. People most naturally take the path of least resistance
and sometimes view that the more healthy
choices require more effort."[8]

—Dr. Ellan Duke, River Hills Chiropractic Clinic

"Poor information is a driver when it comes to people's choices,"[9] says Jonathan Lizotte, Founder of Designs for Health. He shares how we're inclined toward bad decisions because that's what's easy. He feels that we don't make healthier choices because it's hard and we're not willing to invest our time in it.

---

8   Dr. Ellan Duke, interview with author on June 22, 2017.
9   Jonathan Lizotte, interview with author on June 21, 2017.

Can you remember starting a new diet, full of excitement and clear focus on what you wanted? At first it seemed like nothing could stop you from reaching your goal... then came reality. Those first few days of the diet can quickly throw you into shock, as you begin feeling desperate watching your resolve wane as the days grow longer and harder. Your confidence takes a dive as you start questioning how you're going to make it. Willpower has certainly taken many of us far in life, but to depend on it alone would be a mistake.

You see, willpower comes into play in helping you make decisions—whether to stay in bed or get up, whether to eat a cookie or an apple, whether to watch TV or take a walk, whether to stay home or go to work. You get the picture. Willpower is exerted when we face difficult choices, where we're looking at what we *want* to do versus what we *should* do. In many cases, we end up doing what we want to do because we don't see how one million small daily decisions tie into our whole lives and end up getting us where we are going. (Think about that. Where are *you* going?) We don't see those decisions as creating a path down a road we might not really want to take. When we stop and think, that's not really where we want to end up.

> *"If you don't know where you are going,*
> *you'll end up someplace else."*
>
> —Yogi Berra

14

1. The first step in achieving your health goals is to **decide where you want to be**. Once you've made that decision, you'll want to see where the road you're on is taking you. If it's taking you somewhere other than where you want to be, you'd better change course, right? Part of that plan is to start asking yourself questions like "Where will this choice lead me?" If you're trying to lose weight and you know that eating candy is taking you down a road that leads to a place you don't want to go, then you're faced with a choice. Being dishonest with yourself only hurts you. Using questions to get you out of difficult situations is a great way to bring awareness to what you really want. While part of you wants a donut, the other part of you has already decided where you want to go and knows that the donut will take you off that path.

We can see how **willpower without reasoning and clear goals can be difficult**, but even when we've decided what we want, it can be tiring to depend on willpower alone because our brains are constantly working. And similar to working out a muscle, exercising your brain's willpower leads to its fatigue. According to a research performed at Cornell's Food and Brand Lab, we make, on average, about 200 food decisions every day, most of which are not consciously made.[10] How do your decisions usually turn out when you're at the end of a day where you've said no to hundreds of "bad things" and are exhausted and want to give up? I don't know about you, but I usually cave in to what feels good.

> Willpower is exerted when we face difficult choices, where we're looking at what we *want* to do versus what we *should* do.

---

10   Nymag.com, www.nymag.com/scienceofus/2016/05/you-will-make-200-decisions-about-food-today.html (accessed January 22, 2018).

The same research showed that we tend to eat junk food when stressed. We want to give our brains a break, so we're kind of on autopilot. Let's see how an autopilot system plays out in streamlining our decisions.

2. While any change can be difficult at first, beginning change without a solid system is a sure way to fail—and fast. The system I'm referring to drives our decisions, and it works the same for all of us, but its effectiveness in our individual lives depends on the content and soundness of our own system. Here's the system: **Our thoughts and assumptions become our beliefs; our beliefs shape our worldviews, becoming our values that drive our decisions and bear fruit in the form of consequences.** This idea isn't new.

> *"Your beliefs become your thoughts,*
> *Your thoughts become your words,*
> *Your words become your actions,*
> *Your actions become your habits,*
> *Your habits become your values,*
> *Your values become your destiny."*
>
> —Mahatma Gandhi

What goes in must come out, in one form or the other, and we tend to forget these truths and neglect to realize the power that influencers have on us. The diagram below shows how our simplest thoughts and assumptions are the seeds that sprout into choices, which turn into actions that become habits and ultimately bear consequences or produce results. Deciding *not* to take action still has consequences.

"Don't choose at all, and you've made the choice to be the passive receiver of whatever comes your way." [11]

—Darren Hardy

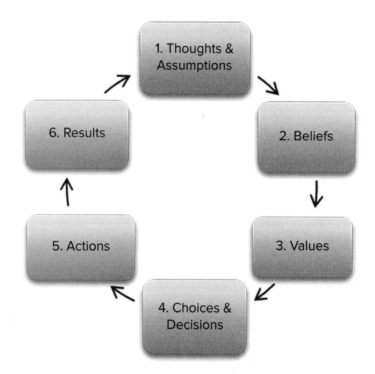

---

11   Darren Hardy, *The Compound Effect: Jumpstart Your Income, Your Life, Your Success* (New York: Vanguard Press, 2010), 23.

*"In essence, you make your choices,
and then your choices make you." "Every decision,
no matter how slight, alters the trajectory of your life."[12]*

—Darren Hardy

Earl Nightingale puts it this way: "Whatever we plant in our subconscious mind and nourish with repetition and emotion will one day become a reality." I also like how Darya Rose, author of the book *Foodist*, explains it: "People whose food choices are driven by their personal values are not lured by temptation because they believe their actions have meaning beyond their own hedonistic desires."[13] Darya goes on to say that their choices are very clear for such people, as they're always consistent with their values. Why do people abide by the Ten Commandments? Because they believe they're accountable to a God who knows best for them, and they understand how following these rules is better for everyone. By understanding all the consequences of harming or even killing another person, I'm better able to make the choice to stay out of these situations without giving it much thought. If in my heart I know something is wrong, I can't justify doing that thing, no matter how I feel in the moment. This concept was examined by a recent study conducted at Stanford University.[14] The students in the study were grouped into two categories: Three-fourths took classes on health and diet, while the remainder studied the food system as it relates to society.

---

12 Hardy, *The Compound Effect*, 23.

13 Darya Rose, PhD, *Foodist: Using Real Food and Real Science to Lose Weight without Dieting* (New York: Harper One, 2013), 303, 304.

14 Hekler, Garnder, and Robinson, "Effects of a College Course About Food and Society on Students' Eating Behaviors," 543–47.

The results were surprising. The students from the food and society class began eating healthier, while the students taking health classes ate less healthily! Why? Because they understood the impact of their choices well beyond their own individual health, as they now considered things like the environment, animal rights, and a healthy diet (what one eats, not restrictions). Can you see how their knowledge impacted their belief system, which, in turn, became a part of their own values, impacting their behaviors?

To better understand the impact of this system, let's visit an economic concept. The concept of "externality" teaches us that *no man is an island*. Just as my choice to smoke affects those around me, the way I choose to spend my money and live my life affects those around me; our collective choices impact the Earth and the course of human history in its entirety. That's amazing! Think about it. If you choose to buy conventional meat because it costs you less, you're discounting its "external" cost and mistakenly believe the meat "costs less." But what you may not realize is that you're supporting the inhumane, irresponsible, and unsustainable conditions in which animals are raised and stimulating industrial farming that destroys our natural resources and poisons us and our planet. "The ninety-nine-cent price of a fast-food hamburger simply doesn't take account of that meal's true cost—to soil, oil, public health, the public purse, etc., costs which are never charged directly to the consumer but, indirectly and invisibly, to the taxpayer (in the form of subsidies), the health care system (in the form of pollution), not to mention the welfare of the workers in the feedlot and the slaughterhouse and the welfare of the animals themselves."[15] Just because you "externalize" the costs doesn't mean those costs disappear. It only means you shift them to someone else (generally your children) and that together humans will end up paying.

---

15 Michael Pollan, *The Omnivore's Dilemma: A Natural History of Four Meals* (New York: Penguin Group, 2006), 200.

Once you understand how that low-quality meat impacts your own health and future as well as the health and future of humans and animals, it should be much easier for you to examine your choices in light of your values and decide if you want to be part of this system, or if you must make alternative choices.

When asked how the American way of life has a negative impact on our health, Gunnar Lovelace, co-founder and co-CEO of Thrive Market, said, "The way we produce food is literally making us sick. Agricultural subsidies dating back to the 1930s were intended to stabilize crop prices, safeguard farming jobs and provide Americans with an affordable and reliable food supply—promoting the production of corn and soy. As farming practices have become more industrialized and efficient, farmers have increasingly sought to produce subsidized crops, ignoring others like vegetables, fruits, grains and beans. We've transitioned as a society with 75% of our modern diet coming from 12 plant species as compared to thousands only 100 years ago. The majority of the food we eat is derived from highly subsidized crops, including high-fructose corn syrup, hydrogenated fats from soy and cheap feed for livestock."

Think about the idea of "voting" with your dollars. Where you spend your money is what you're supporting. If you've picked up this book, I think it's safe to assume you'd rather spend your money on something that's good for you. We all have to eat to live, but would you buy food that is cheaper if you knew it harmed someone else? Think about it this way: Would you buy a pack of gum if you knew it supported terrorism? Most of us would easily answer no to that question, but the problem is that most of us are unaware of where our food and products come from.

Joel Salatin, owner and operator of Polyface Farms, says, *"The average person is still under the aberrant delusion that food should be somebody else's responsibility until I'm ready to eat it."*[16]

Do you understand what you are supporting when purchasing a product, or are you just another consumer who shuffles along, buying whatever pleases you in the moment? Do you ever wonder where your food comes from, who was involved, and how the animals were treated? Do you even know what is in your food? If you saw the list of ingredients in the diet of the cow you're now eating, you might think twice about driving through that fast-food restaurant. Once you know what is important to you, it makes the decision easier and, in a practical way, automatic.

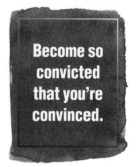

Become so convicted that you're convinced.

Something great to think about from *The Compound Effect*: "How many of my behaviors have I not 'voted on'? What am I doing that I didn't consciously choose to do, yet continue to do every day?"[17]

"The paradox is, as with so many things in life, that the healthier you are, the easier it is to stay healthy."[18]

—Dr. Alan Christianson

---

16   Telpner, *UnDiet, 80.*

17   Hardy, 24.

18   Alan Christianson, NMD, *The Adrenal Reset Diet: Strategically Cycle Carbs and Proteins to Lose Weight, Balance Hormones, and Move from Stressed to Thriving* (New York: Harmony Books, 2014), 176.

You don't even think twice about it. The idea is to **become so convicted that you're convinced**. Conviction is a powerful emotion that usually leads to the formation of our values and beliefs. Once something is a part of our value system, decisions are a piece of cake, as they fall right in line with our beliefs and what we choose to be a part of and choose to remove ourselves from. Of course, it's not a 100% fail-proof system, but it sure beats depending on willpower that will eventually tire and fail. If you think this might not be enough, I'll share more tools in the upcoming chapters to help you overcome your obstacles and meet your health goals.

Josh Gitalis, CN, IFMCP, says, "Health is a continuum. You're either moving toward it or away from it."

So how do you become informed? Reading works for some people (thank you for picking up this book and reading this far!), but for many, it doesn't. Even for avid readers, TV programs and documentaries offer quick, easy, and entertaining ways to educate yourself on a topic, especially for visual learners. For a list of resources to help you build a strong value system and simplify decision making, go to www.leahcampian.com/learning-tools

One year from now, 10 years from now, at the end of your life, when you're asking yourself, "How did I get here?" the answer is very simple: **Just look back at all the choices you made along the way!** As Josh Gitalis, CN, IFMCP, says, "Health is a continuum. You're either moving toward it or away from it."[19] You're either degrading and compromising your health or improving it. In the coming chapters, we'll uncover the

---

19   Josh Gitalis, interview with author on September 8, 2017.

many factors that play a role in where we find ourselves on that sliding scale and particularly how we can get on the upward slope to gaining and maintaining our health!

"Champions do not become champions on the court. They are merely recognized on the court. They become champions in their daily routine. Players do not really decide their future, they decide their habits, then their habits decide their future."

—T. Alan Armstrong

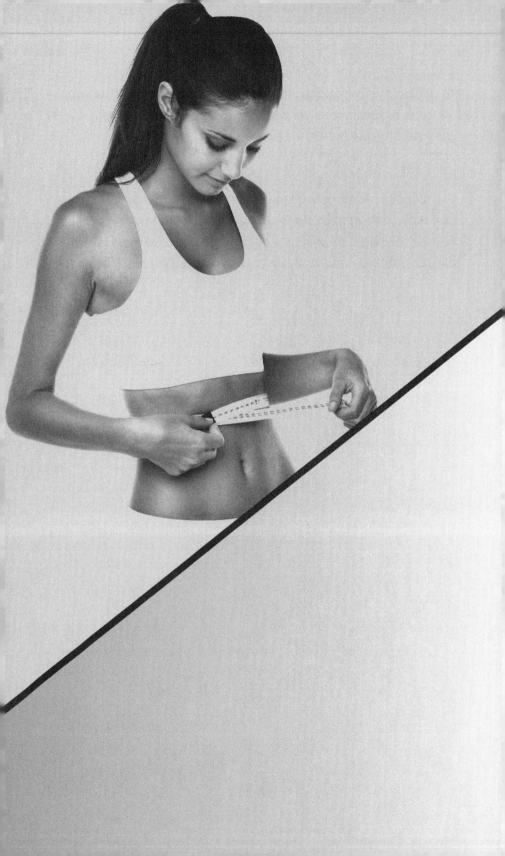

What Doesn't Work:
Counting and Measuring

*"Your relationship with food is yours alone.
It's not like anybody else's. Intuitive eating is not a
food plan, but an opportunity for you to explore your
own reactions to, and experiences with, food."*[20]

—Nan Allison, MS, RD and Carol Beck, MS

20   Nan Allison, MS, RD, and Carol Beck, MS, *Full & Fulfilled: The Science of Eating to Your
     Soul's Satisfaction* (Nashville: AB Books, 1998, 2000), vi.

"[Intuitive eating] is not 'perfect' eating; it is individualized, cyclical, and rhythmic; it includes a wide variety of foods; it is free of obsession; it is nourishing, it feels good, and is an essential component of self-care; it enables participation in life rather than feeling imprisoned by food and our bodies. It is knowing that emotions and body signals, both pleasant and unpleasant, are ways that your body and soul let you know how to care for them."[21]

—Nan Allison, MS, RD and Carol Beck, MS

"Calorie counting is rooted in the assumption that our bodies work like balance scales. Balance scales do not measure quality."[22]

—Jonathan Bailor

I t might be cheesy, but it's true: It's not the counting that counts! Man, was this a hard one for me to wrap my brain around! After so many years of conditioning, it wasn't immediately easy (If I wasn't measuring food or exercise, I was measuring my body; it was nonstop.), but once I tried it, it was so liberating to stop counting and measuring.

---

21   Allison and Beck, MS, *Full & Fulfilled*, 91.

22   Jonathan Bailor, *The Calorie Myth: How to Eat More, Exercise Less, Lose Weight, and Live Better* (New York: HarperCollins Publishers, 2014), 63.

Improve Your Mind-Body Connection

So what's the alternative to counting and measuring? **Learning to listen to your body.**

"Instead of waiting for a health crisis to force us to pay attention to the body, cultivate body wisdom now and learn to work with the body as it changes from day to day."[23]

—Marc David

This isn't something we're big on in our culture, and we're not good at it. Did anyone ever teach you to listen to your body? On the contrary, I had learned to ignore my body and got pretty good at it. With mantras like "No pain, no gain," I was among the toughest. But what good did it do me? Instead of connecting my mind to my own body and staying constantly aware of my needs, I was using external sources to tell me what I needed. How much sense does that make? I have since learned that I am more than a number on a scale, my BMI (Body Mass Index), or the amount of calories I consume, as those are not true measures of my health and well-being.

Just like me, you know a lot more than you think about your own health, more than you give yourself credit for. No one else, not even your doctor, not even me, can tell you what you really need. If you find this hard to believe, you're not alone. In our society, we've lost our intuition—our innate ability to decipher and make the best decisions. But I have good news: We can retrain ourselves by learning to listen to our bodies. It's a skill that takes time, but it's simple.

---

23 Marc David, *Nourishing Wisdom: A Mind-Body Approach to Nutrition and Well-Being* (New York: Bell Tower, 1991), 137.

❖ Find out what the pain, symptom, or craving is *telling* you.

❖ Don't ignore it. Don't jump to end it or quickly satisfy it with what's easy and feels good. Don't look for a pill or cream to treat it.

❖ Rather, **experience** it and let it **guide** you.

As part of a society that encourages instant gratification, we too often look for a quick fix. When it comes to our health, we must learn to understand our body's functions and needs so that we can allow the body to heal itself. We usually look for remedies and cures before understanding the root cause: What caused the problem in the first place? Wouldn't it make more sense to remove the issue instead of just making yourself feel better temporarily, only waiting for it to return again? Think about it: Why do we pull out a splinter before we apply medicine? The same principle applies to your health. Taking antihistamines and steroids for my allergies did help, but once I learned that my eating habits were causing the allergies to worsen, I could change them instead of continuing to take medicine that had side effects and a hefty bill to boot.

Hear me out here. I'm not saying we don't need medical testing or we don't need any medicine ever, but it is amazing how much we've come to depend on these devices. We're putting the burden of our health on someone else instead of taking care of our own selves. In many cases, we can learn that we have high blood pressure based on the symptoms we're experiencing. After all, your doctor knows what those symptoms are, and with his/her help, you can measure your blood pressure and confirm. Once you learn how to change your eating habits and

> A great way to improve our internal instincts is to turn off the background noise.

lifestyle to support better health, you can lower your blood pressure without the use of any medicine. Many doctors are ecstatic to have patients who want to change themselves first before taking medication. If your doctor seems to want you to depend on medication, it might be time to consider finding a new one.

We have access to so much information these days that sometimes we make it a choice of the brain, completely forgetting about our gut instinct. The following excerpt from the book *How We Decide* by Jonah Lehrer reminds us of this fact. "Over time, the brain's flexible cells become the source of expertise. Although we tend to think of experts as being weighed down by information, their intelligence dependent on a vast amount of explicit knowledge, experts are actually profoundly intuitive. The expert naturally depends on the emotions generated by his dopamine neurons... which allows him to tap into a set of accurate feelings he can't begin to explain."[24]

> As part of a society that encourages instant gratification, we too often look for a quick fix. When it comes to our health, we must learn to understand our body's functions and needs so that we can allow the body to heal itself.

A great way to improve our internal instincts is to turn off the background noise. It takes wisdom and courage when there is so much information and overstimulation all around us. While knowledge is power, it can also be overwhelming and quite confusing. Information overload can *paralyze* us. How ironic that the answer at our fingertips could be the cause of *indecision*. We're bombarded with contradicting

---

24   Jonah Lehrer, *How We Decide* (New York: First Mariner Books, 2009), 54.

information. Which voice is louder? There is wisdom in "overriding" science. I'm not saying that you should use that as a cop-out or to say that science is irrelevant or useless. What I am saying is that no matter what you learn or read, no matter what the evidence might show, there are many instances in which science has no power to penetrate and no final answer, so only you can know what is best for *you* if you learn to maintain balance and stay in awareness with your body.

I understand if you're feeling a little confused about all this "listening to your body" talk. Some of you may be thinking, "Well, I've listened to my body and look where it got me!" I'm not talking about giving in to every craving you have, eating mindlessly because you just want to, or sitting on the couch because you don't have the motivation to get up and move. I'm talking about something deeper than a surface-level feeling or emotion. I'm talking about digging deeper and questioning why you have those desires or feelings. When we dig deeper, we can identify the root cause and address that instead of putting a Band-Aid on the symptom and hoping it will eventually go away!

We can also explore other alternatives for meeting our body's needs and desires that might be less harmful than the choices we've made in the past. It's about being aware of what's going on in your body and seeing how your choices play out in your life. How do they make you look and feel? If you can see how your poor choices are tied to your current results and don't like what you've become or where you're headed, you have the insight and power to tweak those choices, one by one, until you get better results. Listening to your body can be easy when you desire something, but the part we most often forget about is to check back in with ourselves and ask and observe how we're really feeling about that

> **There is wisdom in "overriding" science.**

choice we made. Sometimes, we feel immediately good after having a candy bar because of the surge in blood sugar, but later we feel pretty crummy. That's the part we usually ignore. We leave the valuable information unnoticed, simply repeating the same behaviors and choices that keep us stuck in the same undesirable place. In her book *Women, Food, and Desire*, Alexandra Jamieson explains **intuitive eating**: "To eat to honor not just how you feel now, but how you wish to feel two hours from now, three days from now, one month from now, and so on. The goal is to eat in order to live your life to its absolute fullest."[25]

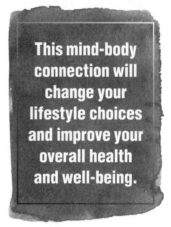

This mind-body connection will change your lifestyle choices and improve your overall health and well-being.

Our minds hold the power to build or destroy, to strengthen or to weaken, yet we have not learned how to use them congruently with our bodies in order to reap the full benefits. We have an untapped power source within ourselves. If I want to see changes in my body but the message in my mind isn't supportive, how's that going to work out for me? Based on my experience, it won't! Stop expecting perfection. Let go of the expectations and empty promises and see what a freeing experience it can be! Once you become aware of your wholeness and completeness, you'll be in awe and have no choice but to honor your body by staying connected to it. This mind-body connection will change your lifestyle choices and improve your overall health and well-being. Now *you'll* decide what to eat and how to move. As you pay more attention to how your body feels, you'll know what foods make you hurt or which ones make you feel good

---

25   Alexandra Jamieson, *Women, Food, and Desire: Honor Your Cravings, Embrace Your Desires, Reclaim Your Body* (New York: Gallery Books, 2015), 129.

and give you more energy. Just listen to your body. Try new things to see what speaks to you. Are you doing something because you heard it was good for you or because *you* want to do it?

Eat Mindfully

You might be wondering how someone could lose weight without counting and measuring what they're eating or how much they're exercising. Let's start with eating. It's quite simple. If you eat more than your body needs for energy, your body may store that food as fat. But the quality of the food is also of utmost importance. Eating 100 calories of sugar or 100 calories of vegetables isn't the same in terms of how your body uses and reacts to those calories. If a calorie is just a calorie, we should get the same results no matter what we eat, but our bodies are more complex than a math problem. You may be eating the same amount of calories, but the results you'll get will be very different, depending on the other components of the food, beyond calories. The solution for those who are eating too much is to eat less by using the body as a means to measure eating.

> When we learn to eat mindfully, we dramatically improve our quality of life and get much more out of our meals.

1. Start by noticing how much you usually put on your plate, and then begin making the portions smaller.

2. You only want to eat until you are about 80% full. Believe me, you won't be hungry. It usually takes at least 20 minutes before we know we're full, and many of us eat so quickly we don't give our bodies enough time to recognize we've had enough, so we just keep shoveling it in. When we eat too much and too often,

we have to retrain our bodies to know when we're truly hungry. Our body's signal that we're hungry comes from the hormone *ghrelin*, but that hormone won't send the signal if it doesn't work properly. When one hormone is out of balance, there are usually a lot more that are out of whack too. As you work to improve your health, your hormones should start working properly too. The body works best synergistically as a whole, so when you improve one function of the body, it usually allows another part of the body to work better as well.

3. Consider *what* is going on your plate. Besides putting less on your plate and eating to 80% fullness, it is just as important, if not more important, to consider the quality of the food on your plate. We're going to cover this in more detail in another chapter, so stay tuned.

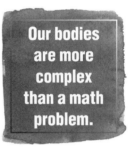

Our bodies are more complex than a math problem.

4. Learn to eat mindfully. I started with the word "learn" because it takes practice to hone this skill over time. So simple yet so difficult for most of us, this skill, once learned, is truly life-altering.

When was the last time you sat down to eat a meal, feeling a sense of gratitude, calmness, unhurried and free to enjoy every morsel, uninterrupted by surrounding disturbances or your own thoughts and feelings? On the contrary, we are often eating on the go, eating so quickly that our digestive system cannot even keep up until we've stuffed ourselves to the point of misery. Then we need a nap, sugar, or coffee—something to get us through the afternoon slump.

When we learn to eat mindfully, we dramatically improve our quality of life and get much more out of our meals.

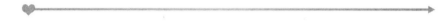

"In a 'me-based society,' we don't gather together and share time as much. Gathering around food allows us to engage, talk, slow down, appreciate the moment, be aware, embrace what's dear. It slows you down and brings you back into balance."[26]

—Justine Kelly, Sun Basket Chef

Here's what mindful eating looks like:

* ❖ It starts with **intention**. Always eat intentionally, not because it's time to eat or you passed by something that smelled delicious. Be sure you're hungry and ready to pause to enjoy your meal.

* ❖ Be fully **engaged** in the choices you make around food, not just reactive. Just because food is placed before you doesn't mean you have to eat all of it or eat any of it.

* ❖ **Preparation** plays a role too. When preparing a meal, think about:
  * where the food came from, how God provided it to us through the Earth, how someone had to work to harvest it;
  * the beauty of the colors, smells, and textures of the food;
  * those for whom you are preparing it, including yourself;
  * how you will enjoy every morsel;
  * how it will provide nourishment;
  * how it will bring people together to bond.

---

26   Justine Kelly, interview with author on June 29, 2017.

- When it's time to eat, all electronic devices and disturbances should be paused. It's not time to watch TV, check emails, send texts, or play games; those will only serve as **distractions**.

- When the food is on the table, pause to **give thanks**, whether in the form of a prayer, verbalized or not. Express gratitude for all the items listed above.

- Once the food is on your plate and you're ready to eat, **pause and take two deep breaths** to clear your mind of any clutter, ready to enjoy the meal that has been prepared. It is very important not to eat when feeling anxious or stressed, as this will inhibit the digestion process and cause malabsorption of nutrients. Taking the time to **get your mind in the right frame** is well worth just a minute of deep breathing to relax and calm you and to make the needed mind shift.

> By bringing awareness to the moment in which you have a meal, you'll automatically begin to bring more awareness to everything else you do in life.

- Use all your **senses**. Look at your food and enjoy how it looks on your plate— the colors and textures. Take the first bite and put down your utensils while you slowly chew the food and enjoy all the sensory pleasures it provides: Smell, taste, texture. You can even close your eyes if it helps you to really enjoy the meal, to start.

- Continue to enjoy every bite, **chewing slowly** throughout the meal, enjoying conversation, yet careful not to eat too quickly while speaking.

❖ At first, count how many times you chew the food, with a goal of 30 to 50 times per bite. Yes, 30 to 50 chews per bite—that's not a typo. Once you've counted for a while, it becomes an automatic response. Chewing your food aids in digestion and nutrient absorption, as your mouth secretes digestive enzymes that begin the **digestion process**. When you've chewed the food well, the stomach doesn't have to work as hard, thus saving your body energy.

❖ When you eat slowly and enjoy every bite, you'll **feel fuller sooner** and will learn to eat only what you need. Remember, the goal is to eat to about 80% fullness. You want to feel energized from the meal, not in need of a nap, which we feel when we've stuffed ourselves.

❖ **True satisfaction** from the meal will help prevent snacking later and even the desire for something sweet right after the meal.

You might be thinking this would be impossible at work, but please believe me when I say your life depends on it! Your health is up to you. Your employer or boss won't see the need to take care of you (nor is it their responsibility) as you must take care of yourself. If you have a limited amount of time to eat at work, make the very best of that time—I urge you.

The reason this practice is so important is that it determines how well you'll digest the food from a meal, how many of the nutrients your body will absorb from that meal, the amount of food you'll eat during that meal, the amount of time between that meal and the next, whether you'll have cravings for something later, the way you might feel toward other people, your responses to circumstances that arise after that meal, and even holding the power to change your worldview. By bringing awareness to the moment in which you have a meal, you'll automatically begin to bring more awareness to everything else you do in life. **Eating mindfully allows for enjoyment and satisfaction, which can prevent overeating, cravings, and binges.**

For more information on mindful eating and your relationship with food, consider reading *Nourishing Wisdom: A Mind-Body Approach to Nutrition and Well-Being* by Marc David. I love his Five Steps of Whole Body Eating[27]:

1. Make a conscious choice to eat.
2. Ask your body what it wants.
3. Eat with awareness.
4. Listen for feedback (several hours or even days after a meal).
5. Release the meal. (No matter what you ate, LET IT GO! This means no regrets or guilt.)

Exercise with Balance

Now let's circle back to measuring our exercise. Tracking progress is helpful, but when we rely on those mechanisms, we lose our mind-body connection; we start listening to something or someone else to drive our actions instead of listening to our own body's wisdom. While we can certainly gain many benefits from exercise, we want to avoid compulsive workouts because we're either punishing ourselves for what or how much we've eaten or we feel it's absolutely necessary to get in that workout to check it off our list for the day, ignoring our body's signs of exhaustion.

Studies, old and new, demonstrate the immense benefits of exercise on both our body and mind, but exercise can also have a spiritual benefit, depending on how and in what form it is done.

---

27   David, *Nourishing Wisdom*, 137.

The best exercise is the one you love, you'll continue doing, and has multiple benefits. For example, working outside in the garden allows you to:

- ❖ connect with nature (Studies show your benefits are increased in natural settings.);
- ❖ get grounded to the earth for more energy;
- ❖ build muscle and long-bone strength when required to lift, dig, or squat;
- ❖ improve circulation and heart stamina (especially with more rigorous activity);
- ❖ improve flexibility with increased movements over time;
- ❖ disconnect from your worries for mental clarity and peace;
- ❖ reduce stimulation of our modern world;
- ❖ feel gratitude for everything around you in nature.

Such "low-key" movement in nature is underrated because we can't measure how many miles we've run, how much weight we've lifted, etc. While you could monitor your heart rate or how many calories you might have burned, being distracted by checking your current status every five minutes or every time an apparatus signals you can be very disruptive to your ability to mindfully stay engaged and aware in the moment, thus reducing the benefits of that movement.

According to Bill Di Stanisloa, co-founder of Farm Life Foundation, there isn't any regimen with natural exercise that when mandatory can cause us to shut down and get rebellious about exercise. He says each person has their own path to natural health. Some will find their way in a routine, while others will flourish following their body's desires in the moment.[28] We all have to establish our own rhythm and accept when the rhythm changes, allowing it to slow when necessary,

---

28   Bill Di Stanisloa, interview with author on June 27, 2017.

then pick back up when our body is ready. What's most important is that you simply move and do it consistently. Have you heard that sitting is the new smoking? It's not that sitting down is bad for you. It's the sedentary lifestyle that gets us in trouble, and research shows that those who sit most of the time and only get a little movement a few times a week are not improving their overall health situation. The negative impacts could include back and neck pain, nerve damage, spinal damage, poor mental health, inflexibility, exercise injuries, bad circulation, and early morbidity. If you're in a job requiring you to sit all day, consider a standing desk where you could alternate standing and sitting, desk exercises, and getting up and moving as often as possible throughout the day. If you fear loss of productivity, these movements can actually improve your productivity by increased oxygen and blood flow to the brain and increased energy levels. Plus, you won't need to reach for sugar or caffeine!

While almost any form of movement can be beneficial, the latest research is showing the greatest impact on your health in these forms of exercise:

- Any form of movement in nature
- Burst or high-intensity interval training for 20–30 minutes, 2–3 times per week
- Eccentric resistance training, once for 10–20 minutes per week, to be paired with any movements listed below throughout the week
- Less strenuous, long-distance activities that you'd consider enjoyable (walking, hiking, bike riding, swimming)
- Yoga—both vigorous and relaxed forms
- Pilates
- Tai chi or qigong

Those are the types of movements or "exercises" that have multiple benefits, giving you something more than the sole opportunity to burn calories.

Dori Thomsen, owner and instructor at Soluna Yoga & Spa in Jacksonville, Florida, shares one of her secrets with us: "Surround yourself with like-minded individuals who listen, support, and care about you." Besides joining a community like her yoga studio, she also suggests an accountability partner, someone who you agree to exercise with, who you're scheduling the time with, and who is willing to take the journey with you. She loves seeing students' growth on and off the yoga mat. "Learning to be patient with yourself in class teaches you to have patience in a long line at the grocery store,"[29] she says.

Sometimes less *is* more. While running has long been a popular form of exercise, I suggest some caution for women involved in any type of high-intensity exercise, especially for long periods of time. Too much high-intensity cardiovascular training can really throw your hormones off, resulting in exhaustion, change in monthly cycles, infertility, low-thyroid syndrome, increased belly fat, etc. I had my own experience with adrenal fatigue, belly fat, and weight loss plateau. The hormones run the show, as we'll talk about in more detail in Chapter 5. Case in point, have you ever watched *The Biggest Loser* on American television? The trainers are always stumped when the contestants worked their butts off to burn a ton of calories and ate a low-calorie diet as prescribed only to plateau on the scales. This goes to show it's not just about calories in/calories out. There are hormonal, mental, and spiritual aspects involved as well. We'll cover those in greater detail throughout the book. The bottom line is that different exercises work uniquely for everyone depending on our stages of life. Ultimately, you have to know your body and do what's best for you.

---

29   Dori Thomsen, interview with author on June 26, 2017.

To get more support and to enhance your skills in these areas, you'll want to check out my Ditch the Diet Program at www.leahcampian. com/ditch-the-diet-program. I'll walk you step by step through each process to implement the right habits for your unique needs so you can take back your health and lose the weight for good.

Scan the QR code for my Ditch the Diet Program.

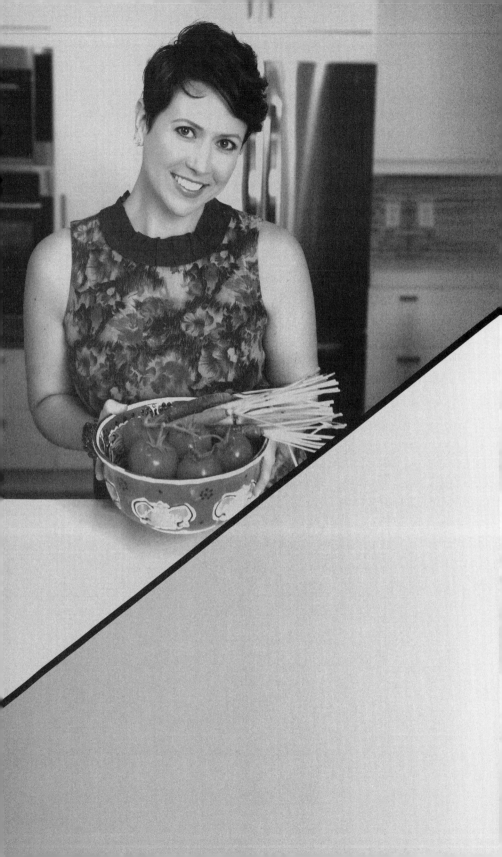

What Doesn't Work:
Focusing on Macronutrients

A ndy Levitt, CEO of Purple Carrot, said, "Understanding food as medicine is pretty compelling."[30] Since being diagnosed with Crohn's disease in 2012, Andy has seen a material difference in how he feels by embracing a whole-food, plant-based diet.

"The influence of technology—phones, television, movies—has blurred what healthy looks like. We're flooded with images of easy, quick, processed foods, enabling and perpetuating a sedentary lifestyle of disease,"[31] says Greg Ferguson, Principal of NaVera Farms. Greg is also a 30-year veteran of the insurance industry, with a keen eye for health care analysis, historical and forecasting trends, and says this type of lifestyle can be seen in medical costs, with an increasing percentage of our population being diagnosed with metabolic syndrome. He says we're living shorter lives that are getting more expensive at the end of our life cycle because of our lifestyle choices.

---

30   Andy Levitt, interview with author on July 18, 2017.

31   Greg Ferguson, interview with author on June 29, 2017.

A big problem I had around food was that I focused so much on the calories, fat, or carbs it contained, overlooking everything else about it, like what vitamins and minerals it had to help me thrive, or how it made me feel, and how my desire for a certain type of food may be a sign that my body is seeking to balance itself, or which foods could be good for me during a needed time of healing. For that reason, sometimes, when I see the words "low-calorie," "low-carb" or "fat-free," I cringe. For so long, that's what I focused on, only to find myself frustrated, never seeing any change. So why does society focus on these factors for weight loss? When I began studying holistic health, I quickly learned that there's a study to support every theory or view, and unfortunately, a lot of studies are being performed to prove a point, not to learn the facts. Now, instead of seeing foods as good or bad and seeing myself as good or bad for my food choices, I know my body well enough to understand which foods will help me to feel and function my best and which ones could cause pain and damage. And that list is ever-changing as I am ever-changing.

Many Americans are obsessed with measuring and glorifying certain macronutrients (proteins, carbohydrates, fats) while shunning others; however, without all of them, we would die. There is no universal right percentage or type for everyone. We all have unique needs that can only be met by carefully listening to our bodies over time and making adjustments throughout the stages of life. I hope that by now you're seeing a theme: **There is no one-size-fits-all solution. We each have to take responsibility for our own health and learn to listen to and understand our bodies individually to make the choices that are best for ourselves.**

"We have more information about what we need in order to have a healthy relationship with food than we've ever had before, but still... we just don't trust ourselves. We still don't trust that we can find our own way with food. And this is what keeps the diet industry alive and kicking. This belief that someone else knows better than we do; that some expert will tell us exactly what to eat, and if we're compliant and obedient, then we'll lose the weight, and then... what?"[32]

—Alexandra Jamieson

Let's take a brief look at each one of the macronutrients and how they're all important to our health.

Proteins

Proteins are made of amino acids that are the building blocks of life, yet our bodies can't make essential amino acids on their own. They must be obtained through food. While meat is a good source of protein, it isn't the only source and may not be the best source for everyone. Some people are better at metabolizing meat than others. While animal sources (meat, seafood, eggs, dairy) provide the best-quality protein, meaning they provide all nine of the essential amino acids or "the right kinds and amounts of amino acids needed to efficiently synthesize our body's new tissue proteins, a variety of plant sources of proteins can do the same job over a period of time."[33] These plant sources include

---

32   Jamieson, *Women, Food, and Desire*, 127.

33   T. Colin Campbell, PhD, and Thomas M. Campbell II, MD, *The China Study: Startling Implications for Diet, Weight Loss, and Long-Term Health* (Dallas: BenBella Books Inc., 2006), 30.

beans, legumes, nuts, seeds, vegetables, and even some fruits. Many people are surprised by how much protein is in plants because they've learned to equate only meat with protein.

Eating a variety of protein sources ensures you're getting all the essential amino acids your body needs, while also providing other vitamins and minerals, and extra fiber from plants to support your health. Keep in mind that without animal proteins, you cannot get enough vitamin B12, which can cause various problems but especially lower energy levels. When consuming meat, follow these guidelines for optimal health:

* Eat **wild-caught** fish and seafood.
* Eat **pasture-raised or grass-fed** meat, poultry, eggs, and dairy products.

Conventionally raised meat, fish, poultry, and eggs are fed antibiotics, hormones or hormone-enhancing substances, fungicides, pesticides, food coloring, and a diet that is usually unnatural to the animal. By consuming low-quality (non-organic, factory-farm raised) meats, you are in effect consuming all these toxic substances as well as the animals' stress hormones caused by inhumane environments in which the animals were raised. Additionally, you'll miss out on the beneficial nutrition superstar omega-3 fatty acids found in the meat of animals consuming their natural diet. As Michael Pollan so eloquently puts it, "The species of animal you eat may matter less than what the animal you're eating has itself eaten."[34]

A note on dairy: It can be a "trigger food" for a lot of people, meaning it can cause health issues. First, I do think it's strange that we're the only beings who continue drinking milk after we've been weaned, not to mention the milk that was intended for another species' offspring.

---

34   Pollan, *The Omnivore's Dilemma*, 269.

This is evident with many of us becoming lactose-intolerant as we age. Besides digestive pain and upset, dairy can be mucous-forming in the body, causing issues like allergies and sinus infections, as well as acne and other skin-related issues. While this can be one of the most difficult ingredients to remove from your diet (Americans love cheese!), it may make one of the biggest impacts on your health. I'd say to give it a try for 30 to 60 days and see how you feel without it. Most people look and feel better. I know I did! I will say that if I consume dairy, it's usually in the form of yogurt from organic, grass-fed cows. I still struggle with eating it regularly, considering the mass production of milk and its effects on the animals and our environment. The dairy cows are pumped every day for most of their lives, often getting infections. By the way, the government allows a certain amount of the pus from those infections in the milk that's sold to you. That gives you something to think about, right? It's best if you know where your milk is coming from so you know how the animals are being treated and what's really in the milk. So go ahead and cry or throw up, but seriously think about it.

Fats

Fats were taboo when I was growing up, thanks to faulty science from the 1950s, but fats have since become more widely accepted among health care experts. That doesn't mean calorie counters aren't steering clear of them! Nor does it mean everyone understands the quality differences of various fats. First, I want to point out that good fat is essential to our well-being and doesn't actually make us fat, contrary to common belief. We all have the ability to absorb fats at different levels, and a fat-free or low-fat diet is **not good for anyone**. Even people with severe gallbladder problems, liver damage, or other medical conditions can usually begin tolerating more fats in their diet once they work to heal their bodies. For an in-depth look at food science, refer to *Death by Food Pyramid* by Denise Minger,[35] or even a lighter read, *Pandora's Lunchbox* by Melanie Warner.[36]

Let's take a look at all the reasons why you want to get plenty of fat in your diet:

❖ Fat is necessary for the **absorption of *most* vitamins and nutrients**. While ***essential fatty acids*** (EFAs) are required in the body, the body can't make them. They can only be obtained through food.

❖ Fat is a major catalyst for **hormone production and balance**; in fact, *cholesterol* is needed to make hormones. (This probably blows your mind because it seems contrary to all that our doctors and drug companies have been telling us for decades!)

❖ Our **brains are 60% fat** and need fat to function properly.

❖ Fat plays an important role in **weight loss**, which might come as a major surprise to you!

❖ Medium chain triglycerides (MCTs) are used as **long-term energy** instead of being stored in the body's fat cells. In fact, they're a longer-lasting source of energy than sugar. Coconut oil is a great source of MCT oil.

❖ Fat helps us to have **regular and healthy elimination (bowel movements)**.

❖ Fat keeps our **skin supple** and our **hair shiny**.

❖ Fat helps us **feel satisfied and full**.

❖ Fat can **decrease inflammation** and **lubricate the joints**.

---

35 Minger, *Death by Food Pyramid.*

36 Melanie Warner, *Pandora's Lunchbox: How Processed Food Took Over the American Meal* (New York: Scribner, 2013).

Quality Matters

What's really important is to focus on the *quality* of the fats you're consuming. Unfortunately, too many "health-conscious" Americans consume too few fats, and the ones we do consume are toxic. The fats used in most processed foods are low-quality, inflammatory hormone disruptors. Those types of oils, derived from the GMO (genetically modified organisms... more on these later) seeds of soy, cotton, corn, vegetables, or canola oils, don't promote health but instead destroy it. Trans fats or hydrogenated oils should be avoided as well.

Learn to identify the healthy fats you want to consume (should be cold-pressed, unrefined):

- ❖ Coconut oil
- ❖ Avocado oil
- ❖ Olive oil – extra virgin
- ❖ Nuts/seeds and oils (except peanuts, as they often contain aflotoxin, a known carcinogen)
- ❖ Hemp seeds and oil
- ❖ Chia seeds
- ❖ Flaxseeds (ground before consuming) and oil
- ❖ Grass-fed butter and ghee (reference my note on dairy above)

Carbohydrates

Of the three macronutrients, "carbs" probably bear the brunt of criticism, but carbohydrates are essential to everyone's diet as a major source of energy and for hormonal balance. "In a study of adults, it was shown that eating under 50 grams of carbs blocked thyroid hormones and caused a 44 percent increase in muscle wasting."[37] The best

---

37   Christianson, *The Adrenal Reset Diet*, 61.

approach to carbs is to first consider consuming only complex carbs versus simple carbs. Complex carbs are foods found in their whole form, without being stripped of other nutrients.

Complex	Simple
Includes whole grains, beans, legumes, vegetables, and fruits	Includes processed food, stripped of naturally occurring nutrients (sometimes added back in but not processed the same by the body)
Requires more digestion, keeping you feeling fuller longer	Requires almost no digestion, leaving you feeling empty
Requires no or little insulin production, helping to maintain a steady blood sugar level	Requires high amounts of insulin to stabilize the blood sugar, resulting in spikes and drops, leading to hypoglycemia and diabetes
Helps to keep us regular	Can cause constipation
Helps weight maintenance and weight loss	Causes weight gain, as what is not used for immediate energy is stored in the body as fat

Fiber is found in carbohydrates, and you need fiber to help with weight loss, remove toxins, and protect your immune system. It's important to consume soluble and insoluble, as well as resistant fiber. While many health experts suggest you stay away from "starchy" carbs for weight loss, *resistant* starches (fiber) can be beneficial for weight loss and general health. They're so called as they "resist" digestion far longer, unlike the other starches that are converted to sugar in our small intestine. They feed the good bacteria in our gut and cause little to no insulin response. While there are many sources of fiber, the best, according to endocrinologist Dr. Alan Christianson, are these three[38]:

- **Resistant**: Boiled potatoes (especially when refrigerated after boiling, like in a potato salad), cannellini beans, navy beans, great northern beans, and unripe bananas
- **Soluble**: Lentils, garbanzo beans (chickpeas), blackberries, flaxseed, and gluten-free rolled oats
- **Insoluble**: Brown rice, quinoa, barley, buckwheat, almonds, broccoli, cabbage, carrots, and potatoes with the skin

Notice that vegetables are an excellent source of complex carbs, yet most Americans are only eating about one serving a day, usually in the form of tomato sauce and french fries! While experts suggest you consume five to nine servings (about half a cup) of fruits and vegetables a day, that number will look different for everyone. Focusing on vegetables is the way to go since they have little to no sugars in them and usually contain more protein and fat than fruits. Eating a variety of vegetables will ensure you get a lot of vitamins and minerals, as well as antioxidants and fiber to help you regularly eliminate toxins from your body. And while most of us don't like the way vegetables taste because we're so used to processed foods, we can learn to make them flavorful to increase our intake over time. More on this later! A great way to think of eating vegetables is to imagine you're eating sunshine! When you consume foods that have been nurtured by the rays of the sun, you're harnessing that same energy for yourself!

Simple carbs, on the other hand, are often referred to as *naked* or *empty* calories. Looking at the chart on the previous page, you can see why, right? These "food derivatives," as I like to call them, are nothing

---

38   Christianson, *The Adrenal Reset Diet*, 55–56.

more than substances that give us temporary energy and fill us in the moment, whether it's to fill our bellies or fuel our brains. Other than those immediate and temporary effects, they don't have the vitamins and minerals our bodies need to support every cell to perform its own function in the body. In other words, they make us sick and we feel pretty bad in the long run. While food companies try to add some of the nutrients back in, our bodies don't recognize those additives the same way they do when the nutrients are naturally occurring in whole foods or in a well-sourced supplement. So even though the label might say that your chocolate chip cookie has vitamin C in it, you can pretty much count on the fact that your body won't be absorbing that vitamin, so it won't be beneficial to you anyway. Let's take a look at why that might be.

"Sugar Is Killing Us"

I'm sure you're aware by now that Americans are obsessed with sugar, but how did we get here? As we moved away from fats, taste in foods had to be derived from *sugar* and salt (sodium glutamates, you might have heard of MSG). Although white refined sugar is bad enough, close to 100% of the processed foods we consume have a much more poisonous substance: High fructose corn syrup (HFCS). Sugar in the form of HFCS is indeed killing our nation, driving unprecedented levels of diabetes, obesity, and cancer. In a recent conversation I had with Dr. Robert Rountree, chief medical officer of Thorne Research, he blamed HFCS as the main cause of the fatty liver epidemic. He said the problem is that it's hidden in almost everything we eat, processed foods you'd never think had sugar in them.[39] Later on, I'll touch more on why this form of sugar is so harmful. For now, let's take a look at the negative health effects of sugar in the forms most Americans consume it.

1. Processed sugar, which has been stripped of its nutrients and bleached in the processing method, provides us with **no nutritional value**, and in fact causes our bodies to work harder to keep diseases at bay.

2. Vitamin C fights with glucose for absorption in the body, so you can see how **sugar "gets in the way."** If you're thinking of drinking orange juice to get more vitamin C when you're sick, be sure there's no added sugar. You'd be better off eating a whole orange, or better yet, broccoli, which has more vitamin C than an orange! Who knew? Just like most of our knowledge, we form our beliefs on what we've been exposed to—*marketing*!

3. Sugar causes major **mood swings, insomnia, sleep disruption, and night sweats**. This is due to its effects on our hormones. Sugar requires high insulin production to stabilize our blood sugar levels. The overproduction of any one hormone throws off our entire hormonal balance, causing a domino effect of symptoms.

4. Those mood swings we experience are due to a drop in blood sugar levels a little while after its initial spike, which causes us to crave it constantly to get back that "high." But that's not the only reason **sugar is very addictive**. If you've ever tried to quit, you know how addictive it can be! It's so addictive it's been compared to "crack cocaine," as it "turns on" the same region

---

39   Dr. Robert Rountree, interview with author on July 14, 2017.

of the brain as cocaine. That's why no amount of self-control or willpower can fight it—*you're essentially fighting against a biological response!*

5. Sugar that isn't used for immediate energy is stored in the body's fat cells, so you can eat all the *fat-free*, sugary junk your stomach can tolerate; it will more than likely **make you *fat***.

6. We've all been told by our dentists that sugar causes tooth decay. So if you want to spend less on dental visits and painful procedures due to a mouth full of cavities, steer clear of sugar! When you do start eliminating sugar, you'll probably see an almost immediate impact in reduced tooth plaque and elimination of bad breath.

7. One last effect I feel I must touch on is that of **acid reflux and indigestion**. Most of us would never associate those issues with overconsumption of sugar or simple carbs because most doctors don't know or don't tell us that it is a major contributor. Here's how it works. The problem is created when we consume so much sugar that it causes an imbalance of bacteria in the gut. Bad bacteria and yeast start to take over the good bacteria in the gut, reducing the amount of acid our stomachs need for digestion. Bear with me. I know this sounds backward, as we've been told we're producing *too much* acid. This lack of acid in our stomachs causes issues when we try to digest meat, which is why we have indigestion. Furthermore, one of the valves that controls access from our stomach to our esophagus gets "lazy" and starts to leak our stomach acid up into our esophagus, which causes the reflux symptoms. So in many instances, contrary to what we've been told, the solution usually isn't antacids or pump inhibitors. Most of us can reverse

these symptoms by eliminating simple carbohydrates from our diets. As we change our diets, using probiotics and digestive enzymes can also help with digestion while we repair our guts.

Now you can understand a little better how sugar is one of the major contributors to a decline in health. While *natural* sugars that have been minimally processed (usually darker in color, like coconut sugar, brown palm sugar, date syrup, unprocessed maple syrup, raw honey, etc.) *do* have nutrients, they are in no way enough to make up most of our diet. Unfortunately, sugar has found its way to the front seat in the standard American diet (SAD). To further understand sugar's role in our diets, I would recommend a couple of eye-opening films: *That Sugar Film* and *Fed Up*. This is part of building your belief system, as mentioned in Chapter 2.

Micronutrients

While macronutrients are vital to our well-being, so are micronutrients. Don't let the name fool you. Though they may be "micro," they are very powerful. **Micronutrients are vitamins and minerals**, and trace minerals (required by the body in amounts smaller than 100 mg) that are essential for our bodies to function all the way down to the cellular level, where we can't see things working behind the scenes to keep us alive and vibrant. Just like the other essential nutrients we've covered, these micronutrients can't be produced by the body and are found in whole foods. To learn more about the role of micronutrients on your health, the book *Naked Calories* by Jason and Mira Calton is a great resource.[40]

---

40   Mira Calton and Jayson Calton, *Naked Calories: Discover How Micronutrients Can Maximize Weight Loss, Prevent Disease and Enhance Your Life* (Howard Beach: Changing Lives Press, 2012).

Micronutrient Supplementation

Supplements can be helpful where there might be nutrient gaps, but theoretically, we shouldn't have to depend on them when our diet and lifestyle are supporting our health. I use some of them on a regular basis and especially during different phases of my life (higher levels of stress, travelling, less access to healthy foods, etc.). I've seen how they've helped me and my clients improve and maintain our health,

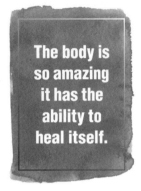

The body is so amazing it has the ability to heal itself.

but we can't rely on them alone. While our bodies were made to absorb nutrients from real food, Dr. Robert Rountree of Thorne Research says that genetic variations increase the need for supplementation in many people.[41] In his practice, he has seen how some herbs and nutritional supplements work at least as effectively as medication but without the undesirable side effects.

The body is so amazing it has the ability to heal itself with our support. Something we don't hear or think much about in this world of abundance in which we live is malnourishment, yet in the West, many of us are overfed and undernourished. This undernourishment is reflected by the many diseases we're facing today in epidemic proportions. So what do we do now? How do we reverse these diseases? A major way of supporting our bodies is through what we put in our mouths. Hippocrates was on to something when he said, "Let thy food be thy medicine." The body can recognize and utilize what it needs, and fortunately, for us, we already have all that we need. When God created us, He put everything in nature that we would need to take care of ourselves. So the real focus here shouldn't be on counting anything. It should be on eating REAL food. A good rule of thumb is this: If it didn't

---

41   Dr. Robert Rountree, interview with author on July 14, 2017.

grow from the earth or doesn't have a mother, don't eat it. That's pretty simple, right? There are a few more details I've touched on above, but if you keep it simple, your body should be able to take care of the rest. It's really about **focusing on the *quality* of calories over the quantity of calories**. When you start eating real food, the more you will want to continue eating that instead of the "junk" you're used to. You'll find that your body knows what to do with the nutrients from real food instead of storing "unknown" substances in your fat cells. You'll start to watch the weight fall off your body without making too much of an effort only by shifting your focus to real food, which is what your body recognizes and truly wants. I understand the cravings for junk food, but that's because your brain has been conditioned by chemicals and the overuse of sodium, sugars, and unhealthy fats (more on that in Chapter 8). In a recent conversation with Dr. Ellan Duke, chair of the Mayor's Council on Fitness and Well-Being in Jacksonville, Florida, she gave the perfect example of this: "Several years ago we mandated that school lunches would be required to include a piece of fresh fruit. In the early stages of this program, it was noted that more than half of these ended up in the trash. Interestingly, **taste buds evolve to appreciate what they are familiar with.**"[42]

Practical Application: When it comes to what you eat, it's best to try a variety of natural foods that are modified as little as possible to get the biggest bang for your buck. Dr. Rountree suggests you develop a new attitude toward food. Instead of fearing it, see it as something with the potential to rejuvenate and nourish you.[43] You'll get the most nutrition out of these foods by learning how to prepare them properly and tastefully. **A very big part of eating should be enjoyment.** If your idea of whole foods is a tasteless salad every day, you're missing out on a lot! When we don't enjoy what we're eating, we're not going to

---

42   Dr. Ellan Duke, interview with author on June 22, 2017.

43   Dr. Robert Rountree, interview with author on July 14, 2017.

stick to a healthy eating plan, no matter how good it is for us! Part of owning your health is learning to try new foods that you might not have been exposed to before, trying to prepare them in different ways until you find something you like. In my opinion, **you should always love what you're eating!**

Enjoying healthy foods doesn't usually happen overnight. It takes patience, trial and error, resolve, an open mind, and a burning desire to make it work! While some of us are naturally better cooks than others, it's a life skill we should all learn to enhance, *whether we enjoy it or not.* I don't particularly enjoy driving, but I had to learn to drive if I was going to get anywhere (not much public transportation where I live). Not to mention that I drive almost every single day of my life, so

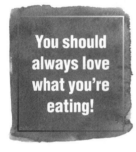

You should always love what you're eating!

I'd say that was definitely a skill worth learning, wouldn't you? Cookbooks give you good ideas for adding flavor to your recipes, which is something so simple yet often overlooked. A bland dish will definitely turn you off and send you running back for processed food, full of toxic, artificial flavoring before you know it!

If you don't know how to cook, aren't very good at it, or don't enjoy it, it's best to start out slowly. If you dive in, you might get overwhelmed and turned off by home cooking. Start by trying a new recipe once a week. Then once you feel you've got that much under control, start to gradually add more until most of what you eat is home cooked. If you have other people in your household, give them a part—all members of the family, young and old, regardless of gender. Everyone should be involved in the process. It will lighten your load, help to create gratitude among everyone, and will help the little ones learn important life skills. On this topic, Dr. Duke shared the following advice with me: "Because we are creatures of habit, it is crucial that we teach our children how to 'make health a habit.' If they see that it was important to their parents, it will be important to them, and hopefully they will pass it along to their children. **This may be the very best inheritance you could possibly pass down.**"[44]

On the other hand, "Eating what's good for you can be hard because other unhealthier choices, like going through a fast-food drive-thru, are convenient,"[45] says Amie Keslar of Front Porch Pickings. She says that because people are busy and tired at the end of the day, they do what's easy. Having been diagnosed with Hashimoto's hypothyroidism, Amie did her research and learned that all autoimmune issues begin in the gut. That's when she decided to begin a whole-foods diet to heal herself. She admits that it can be difficult to get started, but tools like scheduling, meal planning, and food preparation go a long way in making it easier. That's why these tools are all part of my Ditch the Diet Program, to make it easier for you to start and continue! Check out my website for a list of cookbooks and other resources that teach you how to cook with whole foods: www.leahcampian.com/learning-tools

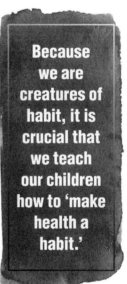

Because we are creatures of habit, it is crucial that we teach our children how to 'make health a habit.'

---

44   Dr. Ellan Duke, interview with author on June 22, 2017.

45   Amie Keslar, interview with author on June 23, 2017.

Scan the QR code for a list of cookbooks and other resources to cook with whole foods.

I will let you in on another little secret that makes a huge difference and makes it easier on you—I would suggest you start adding in the good *before* you remove the harmful foods. Before pulling the rug out from under your feet, look for healthy replacements or alternatives to your current way of eating that isn't supporting your health. Expose yourself to healthy environments and people you might know who eat whole foods. Start sampling some of those foods and try them prepared in different ways. You might not like raw beets, for example, but you might find that you enjoy them in a stew or with other roasted vegetables that are seasoned well. If you don't take the time to find the whole foods you like, you'll be more likely to fail at changing your eating habits. Think about people who give up drugs and replace them with alcohol or smoking. It might be an upgraded choice, in some ways, but we still know the negative impacts of alcohol and smoking on our health. You don't want to stop drinking sodas to reduce your sugar, only to start drinking diet sodas as a replacement, for example. You're just swapping high-fructose corn syrup for artificial sweeteners that can cause cancer and *can cause you to consume even more calories*, leading to weight gain. You're still getting added sodium, citric acid, and artificial colors that can cause neurological problems. My Ditch the Diet Program includes replacements for junk foods and recipes you can start implementing now. To get started, go to www.leahcampian.com/ditch-the-diet-program.

In short, no matter what your eating habits are, at the least, the following guidelines are generally best for everyone. You should consider saying yes to the foods in the left column and eating as little as possible from the foods in the right column. (Note that one column is not necessarily correlated to the opposite column.)

Improving Health	Declining Health
Lots of vegetables, both raw and cooked	Processed foods, especially refined carbohydrates
Fruits (better than juices), including the softer peel if organic	Artificial sweeteners or denatured sugar like bleached sugar or high-fructose corn syrup
Nuts and seeds (best for digestion and nutrition if soaked and sprouted or toasted/roasted)	Non-organic peanuts (butter), inflammatory oils (canola, cottonseed, soy, vegetable)
Whole grains (if tolerated) – soaked/sprouted for nutrition	Denatured grains (bleached), US wheat/barley (contains gluten)
Beans/legumes (if tolerated) – soaked/sprouted for nutrition	Artificial colors, flavors, additives, or preservatives, MSG
Organic when possible	GMO foods; conventional*
Local when possible	Farm-raised fish/seafood
Sustainably sourced meat, wild-caught fish and seafood, pasture-raised poultry, eggs and dairy (if tolerated) – not in excess	Conventionally* raised meat, eggs, dairy, or GMO soy (whether in the form of protein powder, lecithin, tofu, beans...)

*Conventional refers to the standard practice of growing crops or raising animals, which includes the use of herbicides, fungicides, pesticides, antibiotics, growth-enhancing hormones or chemicals.

Wondering how you're going to afford these changes? Think about what Gunnar Lovelace, co-founder and co-CEO of Thrive Market, has to say: "Processed foods traditionally cost less than healthy foods for a number of reasons but primarily due to longer shelf lives and economies of scale. According to a study published in the British

Medical Journal from 2015, eating healthy costs roughly $1.50 more per day than the alternative." It's not really as expensive as we often think it is. For more ideas on ways to save, check out my blog post called "Eating Healthy On A Budget" at www.leahcampian.com.

Dr. Alan Christianson says it's easy to recognize which foods have unhealthy carbs because they come in a box! "Of the 60,000 foods available in American grocery stores, over 80 percent have added fructose and processed carbohydrates. Most foods in the center of the grocery store are some combination of processed wheat flour, high-fructose corn syrup, hydrogenated oils, salt, and artificial flavors and colorings. If something has an ingredient list of more than three to five items, don't bother reading the list; just put it back on the shelf."[46]

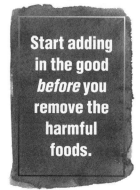

Start adding in the good *before* you remove the harmful foods.

And Jonathan Bailor wrote, "A major reason why we have nutrition labels at all is that much of what we find at the grocery store these days is so far from food that we have no way of knowing its health value without explicit instructions."[47]

With the last two paragraphs in mind, I'd like to warn you about "healthwashing," a term coined by Meghan Telpner in her book *UnDiet*.[48] Before I learned that my body would thrive on eating whole foods, I would pile my shopping cart high with 100-calorie snacks, "healthy" granola bars, microwaveable popcorn, diet sodas, "lean" frozen dinners, fat-free this, and low-fat that. I assumed they were

---

46   Christianson, 61.

47   Jonathan Bailor, *The Calorie Myth*, 162.

48   Telpner, *UnDiet*, 62–63.

> **Foods can harm or help, destroy or support, deplete or give energy; but they don't make you good or bad.**

healthy because of *marketing*! That's it! I simply believed the claims the company was making about the health of that "non-food," based on the label they had used, the advertisements on TV or in magazines, all of which were part of washing my brain to believe they were good for me, all the while wondering why I was still sick and always obsessed with losing weight. So just because a product promises to help you lose belly fat isn't a reason to buy it. Just run it through the criteria listed above, and if it's not real whole food, don't waste your money!

In closing, it's really important you not "label" foods as good or bad, and especially don't label yourself as good or bad for your food choices. Foods can harm or help, destroy or support, deplete or give energy; but they don't make you good or bad. And sometimes, it's not as much the food as it is our own thoughts and behaviors around those foods that determine our ultimate health. (Think about the mindful eating portion in the last chapter.)

"No diet [what one eats] is right or wrong. Any method of eating can provide a deeper nourishment as long as the missing ingredient—consciousness—is present. The ability to reflect on our relationship to food and the awareness that we can expand our perspective on eating at any moment help create the life we want most."[49]

—Marc David (Definition mine)

---

49   David, 176.

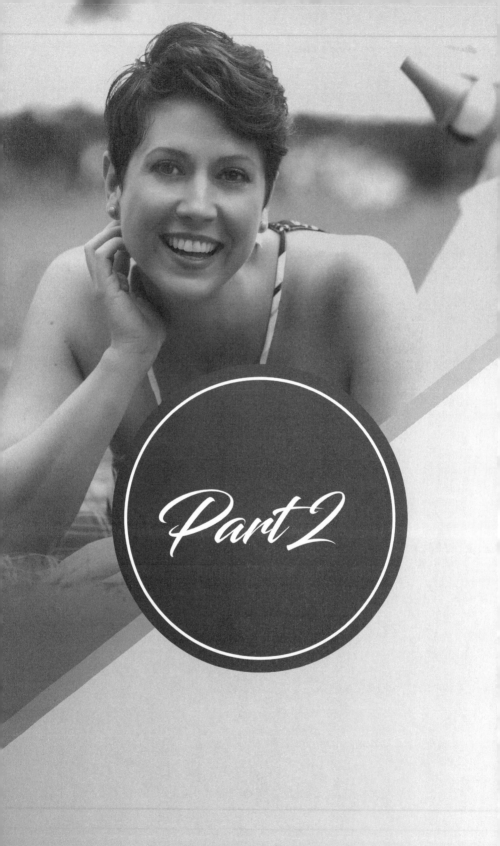

Part 2

Nourishing
YOUR
SPIRIT, SOUL,
AND
MIND

These chapters cover your environment, relationships, toxins, stress, hormones, food addictions, cravings, emotional eating, finding balance, primary foods, fulfillment, your authentic self, purpose, spirituality, soul food, affirmations, new thought processes, the power of the mind, making change permanent, and focusing on the long term.

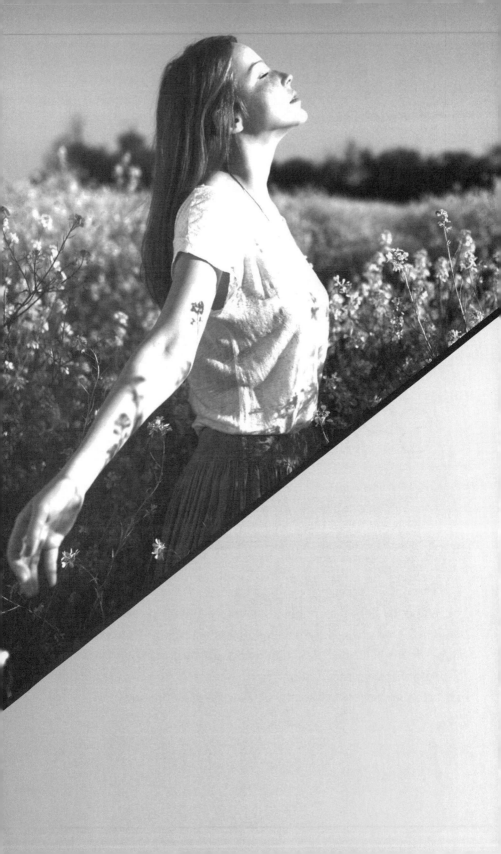

Chapter 5

What Doesn't Work: Environmental Detachment

In my constant struggle to improve my health, something that simply did not cross my mind was how my environment played a role; after all, it was just about the food that came from the market and went on my plate or the amount of calories I could expend in physical activity, but man, was my mind opened when I started researching and learning about what goes into the products we buy and bring into our homes! I'd never thought about what was *in* the food I was eating and in all the products I used on my body, in my hair, in my house and garden. And you might also be wondering why those things matter. While an entire book could be written on this subject alone, I only want to share with you a few very basic items you should be considering so you can take the opportunity to further educate yourself on the subject.

> **Our environment, diet, and stressors can easily throw our hormones out of balance.**

Hormonal Imitators and Blockers

Let's start with a quick look at our hormones and how they "run the show." Our physiology is driven by a closely-knit system of interrelated signals that drive metabolic processes. The messengers that relay signals in this system are our hormones, acting together in an organized way, forming our body's endocrine system. As our body's chemical messengers, hormones drive everything, and they need balance and suitable nutrition to function properly and efficiently. They are totally *inter*dependent, so one could throw off another, if not properly maintained. Our endocrine system also uses neurotransmitters and receivers to send and receive chemical and hormonal messages to our body to perform a particular function. When they're "short-circuited" or are tied up receiving messages from hormone imitators, they don't communicate properly. It works like a lock and key system: If a hormone imitator can fit into the lock, just like the actual hormone itself, the hormone can't get in; it's literally locked out, so communication within our nervous and endocrine systems is inhibited, throwing off our balance and well-being. Dr. Sara Gottfried states the causes of any hormone imbalance include aging, genetics, **poor nutrition**, and/or inadequate "precursors" to make hormones, **environmental exposure** to toxins, **excess stress**, and **lifestyle choices**.[50] The key takeaway is this: Our environment, diet, and stressors can easily throw our hormones out of balance.

So what do hormones have to do with our environment?

❖ Hormonal imitators found throughout our environment, like in genetically modified (GMO) soy and in plastics, to name a few, mimic the hormone called estrogen. When we get exposed to

---

50   Sara Gottfried, MD, *The Hormone Cure: Reclaim Balance, Sleep, and Sex Drive; Lose Weight; Feel Focused, Vital, and Energized Naturally with the Gottfried Protocol* (New York: Scribner, 2014), 49.

them, it's like our body is getting an extra dose of estrogen, throwing off the estrogen balance, wreaking havoc on the entire endocrine system. They've even been linked to cancers of the reproductive organs in recent studies.

❖ Your skin is the body's largest organ, absorbing into the bloodstream 60% of what is put on it and at a rate *faster* than if passing through our digestive system! This makes our skin a vehicle for carrying either toxins or nutrients into our bodies.

❖ The lotions, oils, sunscreen we put on our bodies contain toxic chemicals that build up in our fat cells and can only be released with proper detoxification.

❖ Chemicals called phthalates are in almost anything with fragrances—lotions, perfumes, soaps, shampoos, detergents, deodorants, candles, etc. They make the fragrance last longer but are hormone disruptors.

❖ Even chemicals used in car and furniture upholstery, curtains, and clothing can be detrimental to your health. From causing hormonal imbalances to breathing problems, allergic reactions, and migraines, they are serious promoters of poor health for a lot of people. Most people wouldn't know unless they tried to remove them from their environment.

❖ The Environmental Working Group (EWG) is a great resource to learn about which products are harmful and which ones are safe. They provide a couple of great apps for your smart devices that are very practical, allowing you to scan the barcode of a product to quickly see how it's rated by the EWG.

Harmful Substances and Ingredients

While these substances are certainly influencing our health externally, they're ultimately causing disruptions internally. Take a look at the many harmful substances we're introducing into our bodies orally and how our health is negatively impacted:

- ❖ In an attempt to maximize crop yields, industrial farming makes use of highly toxic **chemical herbicides, pesticides, fungicides, and GMO seeds**, which we then consume when we eat those foods. Long-term exposure to pesticides has been linked to infertility, birth defects, endocrine disruption, neurological disorders, cancer, and more. Some experts say our food supply has become a slow poison to us. To better help you understand GMOs and their impact on your health, I suggest watching the films *Genetic Roulette* and *GMO OMG*. While numerous studies have shown their negative impact on our health, causing many abnormalities and diseases, both short and long-term, no studies have been performed to show their safety in our food! As I write this book, 68 countries require labeling of GMO products and 19 European countries have banned GMOs altogether, according to the Center for Food and Safety. The United States is *not* one of them. (Corn is a GMO crop and full of the poisons listed above. That's why I mentioned in the last chapter how extremely harmful high-fructose corn syrup is to our health.)

- ❖ Studies have linked the consumption of some **artificial ingredients** to cognitive disorders, digestive issues, migraines, neurological problems, infertility, cancers, and other diseases that seem more and more common today. Examples include artificial flavor, food additives, food coloring, preservatives, and artificial sweeteners.

❖ Again, the EWG is a great resource for foods as well. Refer to their list of the "Clean Fifteen" and the "Dirty Dozen" to learn which crops are currently the most likely to have the least and the most pesticides. The list changes every year, sometimes even throughout the year, so it's important to stay on top of current reports for optimal choices and health. Bottom line: Eating organic as often as possible will help reduce your toxic exposure and improve your health both now and later.

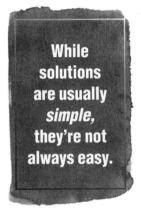

While solutions are usually *simple,* they're not always easy.

Your Skin as a Gateway

Do you or someone you know have skin-related issues? Did you know that these problems often stem from gut and hormonal imbalances? The skin is just showing the symptoms or reactions to an underlying problem going on inside the body. It's natural to look at treating the skin, since that's where we *see* the problem, but remember what we've already covered about holistic health: There's always a root cause, and it takes some time to dig around and find out what's really going on. Here's the good news, though: We can throw our hormones out of kilter when we're not careful of what's going into and on our bodies. By the same token, simple shifts in what you eat and lifestyle can aid the hormones in maintaining balance in our body's systems so we're able to feel and look our best. While solutions are usually *simple*, they're not always easy. Our needs don't often require drastic measures like brain surgery, but lifestyle changes can be very hard to make. There's no need to complicate things, but you have to put in the effort. What's it worth to you?

When asked what consumers should look for in personal care products, Rebecca Hamilton, family owner and VP of Research and Development for Badger Balm, the maker of organic personal care products, gave this advice: "While many companies advertise what they've *eliminated* from their products, they're not always using ingredients that will *enhance* your health." She says that's why labels are misleading. You think it's the best product because it doesn't contain "x, y, and z" ingredients, but what *does* it contain that will improve your health? She suggests you choose products for your skin the same way you'd choose nourishing food. You want something that is naturally rich in nutrients, vitamins, and antioxidants that will be good for your whole-body health, not just for your skin. "Be as close to the source as possible," she says. While you might see olive oil, for example, in a product, cosmetic-grade olive oil isn't the same as freshly pressed extra virgin olive oil because it's chemically extracted, then refined, bleached, and deodorized, leaving it devoid of the naturally occurring therapeutic properties.[51] That's where it comes in handy to find a brand that focuses on providing the best-quality ingredients for you and your family's health.

Toxic Relationships

Another part of this lifestyle shift you will have to make is taking a look at the people and elements of your surroundings. A toxic relationship can have a similar impact on your health as ingesting poison. In fact, the stress caused by a bad relationship has been linked to poor health, manifesting itself through diseases such as IBS (irritable bowel syndrome), stomach ulcers, high blood pressure, cardiac issues, diabetes, and even cancer. If that isn't a motivator for maintaining good, healthy relationships, I don't know what is! Just as your relationships should be supportive of your health, your surroundings should as well.

---

51   Rebecca Hamilton, interview with author on July 26, 2017.

While you should be careful of who you let into your surroundings, you should also make your physical surroundings aesthetically pleasing, free of clutter, and turn them into an element that will motivate you to be your best. It's not something we often think of as being related to our health, but studies show that it is a major driver. If you're allergic to dust and you only dust three times a year, do you think there could be a reason you get chronic sinus infections that make you feel too tired to do anything? If you hate what you see every time you have to go to work, what can you do to improve that environment? The way we feel about our environment consciously and subconsciously influences the way we feel about ourselves, others around us, our life, our circumstances, etc. Having a negative outlook on life isn't going to motivate us to do anything good for ourselves.

While most of this book is focused on changing the inside in order to see results on the outside, this chapter reminds us that the external can have a far greater impact on our health than we ever imagined it could. As you build your system (as covered in Chapter 2) and develop it through exposing yourself to truths like these, you can begin making radical changes to your lifestyle, at your own pace, which will determine the rate at which you'll begin seeing results. It won't be easy, but will certainly be worth it when you begin seeing results. In my Ditch the Diet Program, I share with you great resources to upgrade your lifestyle, as we focus on helping you detox your life, from the inside out, in order to see faster results! While it varies for everyone, most people who have made radical shifts in their environment in a short period of time usually see results as soon as a week from making those upgrades!

To get started making immediate changes in your environment, check out my 21 Day Transformational Nutrition Cleanse at http://www.leahcampian.com/21-day-transformational-cleanse.

Scan the QR code for my 21-Day
Transformational Nutrition Cleanse.

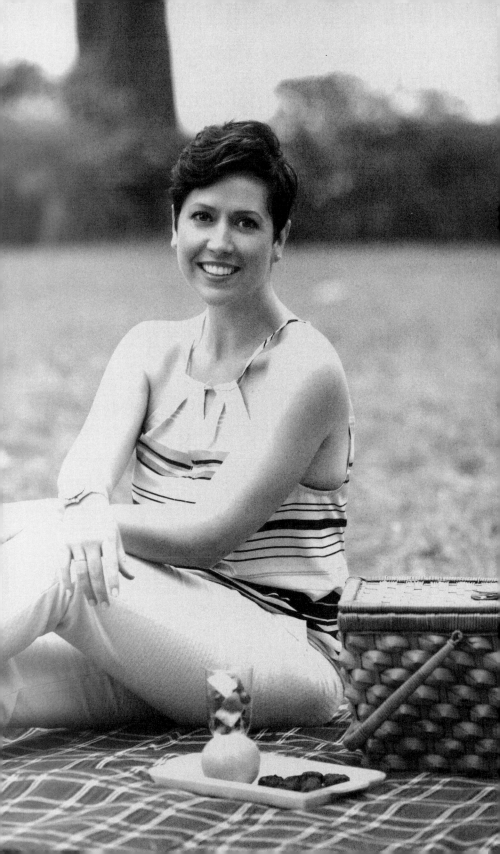

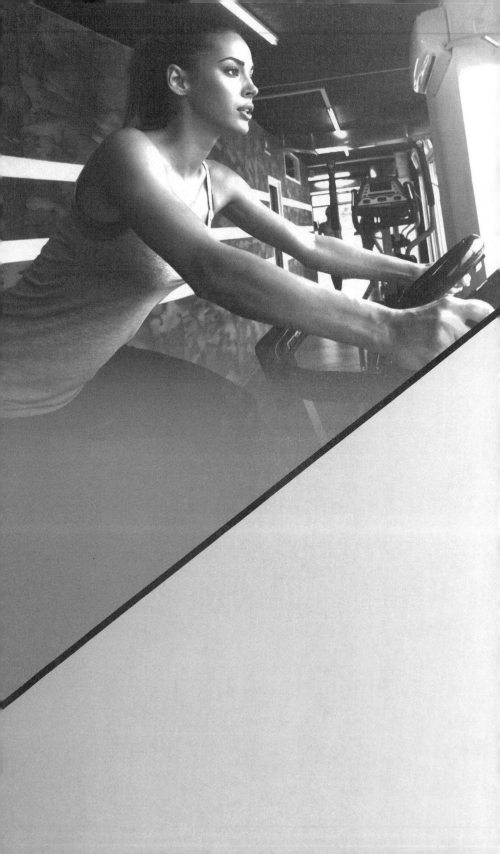

Chapter 6

What Doesn't Work:
One-Dimensional View of Health

When you think of a healthy person, what comes to mind? For most of us, we would see a thin person, all sweaty from working out, with a towel wrapped around their neck, eating an apple. Does that sound about right? When you see that image, where is the focus? It's on *the body*. But is that all health is? For most of my life, I associated my health with my body, and that's it. That blind, narrow-minded view caused me a lot of frustration, wasted energy, extra effort, pain, and suffering. Maybe you find yourself in that same place now. It's very easy to end up there with all the messages we're fed through mainstream media. And remember, if that's your only source for building your belief system (referenced in Chapter 2), the cycle that produces your results is more than likely going to take you somewhere you don't want to end up.

So if our health isn't one-dimensional, how many dimensions are we talking about here? I think the question "Who are we?" holds the answer. We are a three-dimensional reality, are we not? We are mind, body, and spirit (soul). If that's our reality, then it would make the most sense to base our health on all three dimensions to see success, wouldn't it? Furthermore, all three must be in sync for the whole to work. They're truly inseparable and work together to keep us at our best. To separate them would be like cutting off one of your legs and trying to run! It just doesn't make sense, yet we see people striving to be healthy with a one-dimensional focus on the body alone.

While in future chapters we'll delve into the specific ways we can support our mind and spirit, since those are the two dimensions often overlooked, here I want to introduce you to the concept of "primary foods." To have good health, we do need to keep our focus on nourishment and expand the concept beyond our traditional understanding. One definition of **nourishment** is *the food or other substances necessary for growth, health, and good condition.* To receive nourishment, one must be fed not only "ordinary food," like what you eat from a plate, but also what Joshua Rosenthal refers to as **primary food**. Joshua, author of *Integrative Nutrition* and founder of The Institute for Integrative Nutrition, says, "Sometimes we are fed not by food but by the energy in our lives. These moments and feelings demonstrate that everything is food."[52]

Primary Foods

To grasp the idea of primary food, think about what you're "hungry for" in life. What do you crave or desire? Is it play, fun, touch, romance, intimacy, love, achievement, success, art, music, self-expression, leadership, excitement, adventure, belonging, or a spiritual connection? All of those are examples of essential or primary forms of nourishment. While we must eat "ordinary food" to sustain our bodies, the problem

---

52   Joshua Rosenthal, *Integrative Nutrition: Feed Your Hunger for Health & Happiness* (New York: Integrative Nutrition Publishing, 2008), 142.

often lies in replacing our primary nourishment with this secondary form of nourishment we call food. We can see this in our behaviors of stuffing ourselves with food when we feel lonely or hurt, when we're in a job that's unfulfilling or in a relationship that's missing love, or even when we're not getting enough physical movement in our daily lives. While it can take some time to explore the primary foods and fill the gaps, you can at least start by identifying these foods for yourself. Consider how well you're doing in each of these areas and which ones could use some extra attention in your life:

- Overall health
- Physical activity
- Home cooking
- Home environment
- Relationships
- Social life
- Creativity
- Spirituality
- Confidence
- Education
- Career
- Finances

When you assess each area of your life, what's missing? Where do you feel the pain? What can you do to turn that pain into joy? It takes time for introspection, reflecting on the things that have limited you in certain areas, and exploring how to get back your passion where it may have fizzled out. We'll touch more on this in the next chapter.

I hope this list helps you get a better idea of how focusing only on the body or "ordinary food" can limit your growth and health. When I look back at my dieting days, I remember the sole focus being on the external.

I was always comparing my body to my sister's or friend's, or even worse, a model's body. If the comparison of our bodies wasn't the focus, it was the food that haunted me. I had this restrictive mindset that I was only "allowed" to have certain foods. When I saw my skinny friends eating whatever they wanted, I looked on in envy. The way I felt was driven by the food choices I made. If I ate "good foods" that were allowed on my diet, I felt that I was a good person, but if I ate "bad foods," I felt like a failure and ashamed of myself. I would even start judging others who I knew were dieting based on their food choices! This external focus never helped me. It only hindered me. It caused jealousy, self-hate, or pride—none of which served me or those around me.

Once I started focusing on the internal, though, things completely changed for me. Instead of trying so desperately to fit in, I started embracing my own uniqueness. And women, let me tell you, there is nothing more attractive to a man than a woman who is confident in her own skin. If you can't love yourself for who you are, you'll find it very difficult to receive love and acceptance from others. While you may seek it from others, you never really accept it, so it's a futile search that's always going to let you down. As you begin to shift your focus inside and love yourself for who you are, you will be able to see that a part of loving yourself is accepting that certain changes will make you a better version of yourself, so your striving to improve has a whole new view and purpose! **Instead of forcing yourself into another diet because you hate yourself, you instead love yourself enough to see certain food choices and lifestyle changes worth the investment in yourself.** What a freeing mental shift!

Balance

"While technology has helped to increase our productivity, it's also distracting. We need to carve out time in our lives to be disconnected," says Rick Stollmeyer, CEO of MINDBODY. He says we should continually seek to create balance in these four areas he calls "the four Rs": Responsibilities, relationships, recreation, and rest.[53]

One of my greatest challenges is to help people understand that you can't really have it all. We've been conditioned to believe in this illusory "perfect world." Many dream of a family and having "the big bucks" so they can have a lot of stuff they don't really need, a wife who is sexy, thin, educated, successful, has dinner on the table every night, the house and kids clean, and involved in every extracurricular activity available. How can this be possible? In reality, it's not. However, if you come to believe it is and begin chasing the delusion, do you wonder why you're exhausted, depressed, and lack meaningful human connections? With parents like that, do we wonder why our children (who have more opportunities than any other generation in history) are getting sicker younger, are stressed, overwhelmed, and diagnosed with all kinds of behavioral issues? Just the mere attempt of trying to juggle it all creates imbalances, burnout, and overwhelming expectations that cause anxiety and depression.

Instead of looking for the "easy button," look for the "reset button." Stop and think. Reevaluate how realistic your expectations of yourself and others are. We're forced to prioritize because we simply can't have it all. Go back to Chapter 2 and recall your own inner values. Then you can make choices based on what you've already decided is important to you, not based on the outside voices that are pushing you to be the impossible, do the impossible, to the point where the "impossible"

---

53   Rick Stollmeyer, interview with author on July 21, 2017.

negative consequences become real. By impossible consequences, I mean things happening that you never thought could or would happen to you. When we push ourselves beyond our physical limits too often, problems begin to manifest themselves. Once again, you can see how health isn't as much about food as you may have previously thought.

Stress

Let's take a look at your body under stress, just to see how much it impacts our health. First, it's important to understand that *stress is natural*. As a matter of fact, the word *eustress* means "good stress," the kind that motivates us to take action. *Distress*, on the other hand, is the type of stress we find ourselves in too often, unable to manage it, watching it wreak havoc on our health over time. In his book *The UltraMind Solution*, Dr. Mark Hyman says that "Ninety-five percent of disease is either caused by or worsened by stress."[54]

Your Body under Stress

* ❖ Stress is our body's physiological response to perceived danger. It turns on our **sympathetic** nervous system, the fight or flight response, pumping out epinephrine from our adrenal glands and cortisol, which raises our blood sugar levels and blood pressure to get us out of the situation. While this is a natural mechanism, its overuse can be detrimental.

* ❖ **Cortisol** is actually needed in higher levels earlier in the day to get us going then wanes off in the evening so we can sleep, but if it's in high gear at night, trying to help our bodies handle stress, we won't sleep. Its overproduction can also cause excess belly fat.

---

54 Mark Hyman, MD, *The UltraMind Solution: The Simple Way to Defeat Depression, Overcome Anxiety, and Sharpen Your Mind* (New York: Scribner, 2007).

- And after a **surge of glucose** released by the liver, our bodies start pumping out insulin to maintain our blood sugar levels. When we later hit a blood sugar dip, we need to replenish the loss, so what do we go for? Anything that will give us immediate energy: Sugar, caffeine, or both! This creates a cycle that I'm sure many of us are familiar with.

- Once we've escaped the danger that ignited the distress in the first place, the body seeks balance. That's when the *parasympathetic* nervous system kicks in, in what we call the *rest and digest* phase, but only if we allow it to happen. After surviving an "episode," I can hear our bodies say, "Whew, we survived another attack!" Many of our days are consumed with putting out fire after fire, and we don't give our bodies the chance to rest.

- As you can imagine, attack after attack will soon put the body into a state of adrenal fatigue, where it can no longer respond properly to stress. You might feel sluggish, lack energy, and feel unmotivated. This **adrenal fatigue** can also cause other hormonal imbalances, which could lead to **low thyroid**, where our metabolism slows down and we experience dry skin, loss of hair, loss of motivation as well as **infertility**, just to name a couple of consequences of hormonal imbalance.

- Not only do we wear ourselves out, putting ourselves in the worst position to make the best nutrition choices, but when we suffer stress, we can experience indigestion, an upset stomach, bloating, diarrhea, and even malnutrition when we don't allow the body to "rest and digest." Think about it. When you're trying to run from a tiger, all of your energy is focused there. Blood pumping from the heart, to the legs and arms, helping you run faster, and in our current-day situation, it sends messages to our brain to focus on solving the problem, not digesting food. So even the "healthiest eater" will have health issues if their body isn't able to assimilate the nutrients they consume!

In her book *The Hormone Cure*, Dr. Sara Gottfried lists these top seven health risks to high cortisol levels[55]:

1. Abnormal blood sugar, diabetes, and prediabetes
2. Obesity, increased body fat, and metabolic syndrome in women
3. Mood and brain problems, including depression, Alzheimer's disease, and multiple sclerosis
4. Delayed wound healing
5. Infertility and polycystic ovarian syndrome
6. Worsening sleep
7. Bone loss in menopausal women

At this point you may be thinking, "I've *got* to manage my stress levels!" And I couldn't agree more! Here are some helpful guidelines to get you going.

❖ **Reevaluate *every* decision and commitment** you've made, then prioritize them according to your value system. If they don't rank high enough on your valued items, scratch them off!

❖ **Learn to say "No, thank you."** Overcommitting is a big cause of stress!

❖ **Make plans and preparations.** This is especially important when it comes to nourishing ourselves in all ways: Food, movement, spiritual practices, self-care. **Be proactive, not reactive.**

---

55   Gottfried, *The Hormone Cure*, 86–87.

- **Know your triggers** and try to avoid them or learn how to respond to them. More on this later.

- **Become part of a community.** I love how Dr. Alan Christianson says that "interacting with people is every bit as medicinal as broccoli and push-ups." Based on studies done since the '50s and '60s, he concludes that one of the best ways to deal with stress is to focus on someone else's! He shares Dr. Allan Luks's term of the **"Helper's High,"** stating that "those who regularly assist others are ten times more likely to be healthy."[56] Andy Levitt, CEO of Purple Carrot, attributes part of his health improvement to a solid support system from friends and family, as well as a sense of community he gains from participating in group exercise, like spinning classes.[57]

- Incorporate **mindfulness practices** such as prayer, meditation, deep breathing, yoga, tai chi, and qigong to help bring more awareness, balance, peace, and energy into your life. Just 10 minutes a day can go a long way! Rick Stollmeyer of MINDBODY says, "Mindfulness is a dimension of emotional intelligence and must be continually developed over time. A regular meditation practice helps to make us happier, more focused, more effective. It's becoming more widely adopted in Corporate America, where the results are showing more creativity and productivity in employees."[58]

- **Get grounded** by walking barefoot on the beach, gardening, lying on the ground and looking up at the clouds or stars, etc. By coming into close contact with the earth, we receive more of its energy and can find it to be a peaceful experience as it grounds

---

56   Christianson, 184.

57   Andy Levitt, interview with author on July 18, 2017.

58   Rick Stollmeyer, interview with author on July 21, 2017.

us when we're overstimulated by all that's going on around us. This works best if there's nothing between you and the earth (shoes, towels, mats, etc.).

❖ And finally, for the type A personality, **don't sweat the small stuff!** I know that's so much easier said than done, but it all starts with knowing your purpose and values, keeping an open mind and curiosity about life, embracing each experience as an opportunity for life to teach you, and consistent practices that allow you to explore who you are and allow you to express yourself.

Believe me, I get it. It's not possible to completely eliminate stress. I still struggle with it most days, but it's the ability to make gradual and sometimes drastic shifts in our lives that will support our health and make all the difference in our ability to reduce and manage our stress levels. As Robb Wolf reminds us in his book *Wired to Eat*,[59] we have a lot more control over stress simply by learning to shift our *perceptions* of particular situations. He references a practical resource on TED Talk by psychologist Kelly McGonigal, titled *How to Make Stress Your Friend*. I've experienced a shift in my own stress levels and reduced my sense of overwhelm and anxiety simply by learning to adjust my paradigm of previously perceived stressors. Josh Gitalis, CN, IFMCP, advises his patients to adopt consistent stress-processing activities to help move stress through the body.

> It involves a regimen that starts with slowing down, stepping away, making an assessment, then making plans to take action based on discovered needs.

---

59   Robb Wolf, *Wired to Eat: Turn Off Cravings, Rewire Your Appetite for Weight Loss, and Determine the Foods That Work for You* (New York: Harmony Books, 2017).

He suggests activities like yoga, meditation, or light exercise and highlights the importance of continuing them even though they might be difficult at first and you may not see immediate results.[60] Anything new is hard at first and takes repetition to see improvement.

One key piece in your ability to maintain balance throughout life is to begin a self-care regimen. Kristy Alexander, founder and owner of Apple Rose Beauty, says that self-care starts with being aware of every aspect of yourself—mind, body, spirit—so it becomes very personal for each individual. She says it's a way to check in with yourself to really understand where you're lacking and what needs attention. "It involves a regimen that starts with slowing down, stepping away, making an assessment, then making plans to take action based on discovered needs."[61] Kristy takes a "cell phone detox" every week, from 6:00 p.m. Saturday to 6:00 p.m. Sunday so she can give herself the time she needs to disconnect from the noise and reconnect to herself and her personal needs. That time can also be spent with others, but it really depends on what you feel is going to be energizing and restorative to yourself as a whole.

"Meals are the foundation of self-care. Harness the power of each meal to energize, stabilize, and fuel you."[62]

—Lisa Powell, MS, RDN, Director of Nutrition at Canyon Ranch

---

60   Josh Gitalis, interview with author on September 8, 2017.
61   Kristy Alexander, interview with author on July 6, 2017.
62   Lisa Powell, interview with author on June 29, 2017.

In *Wired to Eat*, Robb Wolf says it's just as important to build a community through cultivating relationships. "Numerous studies have shown that inadequate social support, simply lacking meaningful relationships with other people, may be as harmful to our health as a pack-a-day smoking habit."[63] Oxytocin is a hormone often referred to as the bonding or cuddle hormone, as it's produced when we hug a loved one (including pets), when a mother nurses her baby, when we share time with each other bonding. It's a "feel-good" hormone that's an important part of our coping mechanism. When we don't invest the time to develop good relationships, we miss out on the opportunity to reach out to someone for support. At the same time, we can't be of support to others, which helps to improve our own sense of well-being.

As we've moved through this chapter, I hope you can see where we touched on a few of the primary foods, and now you can better understand how to truly nourish yourself by these means *before* turning to "secondary foods" to fill the voids. Seeking balance in each area is key to obtaining and maintaining optimal health. Now let's take a deeper look at meaning by digging a little deeper into the dimensions of the spirit and learn more about what self-love looks like. Chapter 8 will cover more on the mind.

To take a free self-care assessment and receive a comprehensive list of specific ways to practice self-care, go to www.leahcampian.com/self-care-quiz.

---

63   Wolf, *Wired to Eat*, 129.

Scan this QR code to take my self-care quiz to receive your FREE assessment and tips for better self-care! (Valued at $45)

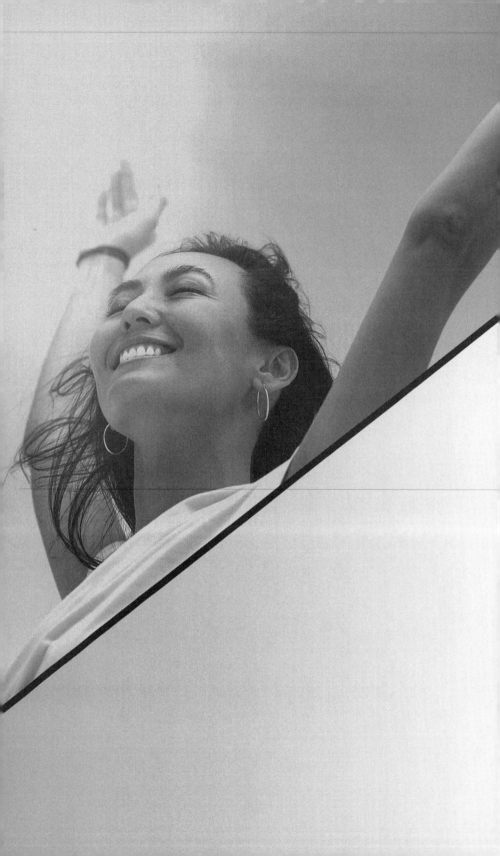

Chapter 7

What Doesn't Work: Meaningless Efforts

"If we fail to understand how to fill our souls with spiritual nourishment, we will be triggered to numb our longings with temporary physical pleasures. When those pleasures are food, the resulting behavior is what we often hear referred to as 'emotional eating.' But this issue is bigger than emotions; it's really about spiritual deprivation."[64]

—Lysa Terkeurst

In the last chapter, we saw that an integral part of our health and overall well-being is tied to our spirit or soul, and just as our body must be fueled to function properly, our soul must be well fed to allow us to thrive. Just as each of our bodies requires a unique diet (eating habits) to meet our individual needs, different things fill our individual souls.

---

64   Lysa Terkeurst, *Made to Crave* (Grand Rapids: Zondervan, 2010), 129.

Define Your True Identity and Purpose

Have you ever wondered who you really are and why you're here now? I believe in a Creator who designed my unique purpose here on Earth. After all, who creates something that serves no purpose at all? If only to entertain you or to make you revel in its beauty, it still has a purpose. I want you to know you were made for more than just a mere physiological existence. You might be thinking, "Who cares if I have a purpose or not?" While I love the willingness to think outside the box and not be constrained or defined by anything, I believe that much frustration comes from feeling a lack of purpose. You see, this is the very thing that drives us on our journey. Moving through the motions of life without purpose is like having a ship with no rudder to guide it in the right direction. Whether we want to admit it or not, we all have this intrinsic longing, this craving. I love how Lysa Terkeurst puts it in her book *Made to Crave*[65]:

> **Just as our body must be fueled to function properly, our soul must be well fed to allow us to thrive.**

"Food can fill our stomachs but never our souls. Possessions can fill our houses but never our hearts. Sex can fill our nights but never our hunger for love. Children can fill our days but never our identities."

---

65 Terkeurst, *Made to Crave*, 64.

"I think a lot of us try to get filled up with things or people. I walked around for years with a little heart-shaped cup, holding it out to other people and things trying to find fulfillment. Some of us hold out our heart-shaped cup to food."[66]

I believe we all have a longing within us that only God can fill. As Brennan Manning states in his book *Abba's Child*, "God created us for union with Himself: This is the original purpose of our lives. And God is defined as love."[67] You see, when you understand that last statement from Scripture, you can see yourself in a whole new light. If we are to commune with God, who is Love, we must accept this love, for others, yes, but for ourselves as well, which can sometimes be the most difficult of the two. To learn more about yourself, it helps tremendously to see yourself through the eyes of the Creator of the universe. Now let's take a deeper look at our identity.

Have you ever felt like you were living out someone else's life? Maybe you would answer no to that question, yet most of us aren't living as our authentic selves. It's actually our ego that's been driving the show most of our lives. Your ego is who you've been conditioned to be, based on fears, desires, what others have influenced you to be, or what you believed you *should* be. Your authentic self, on the other hand, is who you *really* are, deep down, usually hidden behind the ego. Your authentic self gets crowded out by confusing messages over time. By not seeing ourselves through God's eyes, we're disconnected from our true selves, from what He created us to be. Seeing ourselves through God's eyes completely changes the way we see ourselves. Otherwise, we start to believe the lies our ego tells us, that that's who we really are or have to be. So how do we know who we really are? Brennan Manning says, "Define yourself radically as **one beloved by God.**

---

66   Terkeurst, 114.

67   Brennan Manning, *Abba's Child* (Colorado Springs: NavPress, 1994), 50.

This is the true self. Every other identity is illusion."[68] That's a bold statement, but what if you were to just "try it on," see how that feels, and accept it as truth? If God Himself loves you, you can only accept His love by loving yourself. To not love yourself and accept yourself as you are, you are not accepting His love. Try to start by loving who you see in the mirror, even if you know you're not living up to your potential right now. If you're wondering how you love yourself if you don't even know who you are, start by looking at the good, the bad, and the ugly. Don't hate the bad and ugly. Just recognize it as part of yourself and try to understand why that might have come to be a part of you. Love and accept yourself, especially the imperfections (physical or not). It's what makes you so unique and gives you perspective that's not exactly like anyone else's. True love is accepting yourself as you are but desiring the best for yourself too. Sometimes that means change is necessary to live up to your potential.

Learning to be your authentic self involves a spiritual journey. Everyone's spiritual journey is different—unique to oneself. Embarking on a spiritual journey involves a sense of wonder, open-mindedness, acknowledging God in everything around us, accepting life as a teacher, unity with and love and respect for all living beings. How is *your* spirit connected to the spirit of others, to all beings, to nature? They will act as a mirror, showing you things about yourself you never knew or didn't really pay too much attention to before.

Once you've begun examining who you are and begin your spiritual journey, you are in a place to ask God to help you transcend your ego, so the true you can shine through! The ego is there to "protect" us, but if we're not able to rise above it, we can't grow. Being aware of the ego's existence allows us to acknowledge what it may be teaching us but not be bound to it. In letting it go, "keeping it in its place," if you

---

68   Manning, *Abba's Child*, 59.

will, we have the freedom to explore who we really are. To experience self-discovery and inner growth, you have to wonder, be open, be guided. Answers can't come into something or someone who is closed.

One important aspect of spirituality is to just "be." That can be challenging in today's constantly moving world. All we hear is do, do, do; go, go, go! Being still allows us to listen—listen to what our soul is telling us, to what God is teaching us, through the universe He created and through others. I like Brennan's perspective: "While the impostor draws his identity from past achievements and the adulation of others, the true self claims identity in its belovedness. We encounter God in the **ordinariness of life**: not in the search for spiritual highs and extraordinary, mystical experiences but in **our simple presence in life**."[69]

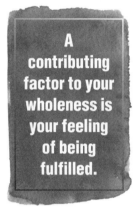

A contributing factor to your wholeness is your feeling of being fulfilled.

Find Fulfillment in *Primary* Food

Let's come back to primary food to see how it fits into the discussion. A contributing factor to your wholeness is your feeling of being fulfilled. We express ourselves through our spirit, which is just as unique as our bodies. Don Miguel Ruiz, author of *The Four Agreements*, says, "Our biggest fear is taking the risk to be alive and express what we really are."[70] Here's how you know when you've found your *primary food*, something that fulfills you: You could do it for hours without feeling tired, sometimes forgetting to eat or drink, because you are so immersed in it, deriving so much pleasure that you don't need anything else at the moment.

---

69   Manning, 50.

70   Don Miguel Ruiz, *The Four Agreements* (San Rafael: Amber-Allen Publishing, 1997).

❖ Try different things and see what moves you and allows you to express who you truly are, not what you've told yourself you have to be or what others believe you are or should be.

❖ It could be reading, writing, cooking, singing, playing an instrument, dancing, drawing, painting, creating something new, sculpting, tinkering with gadgets, any form of movement, teaching, mentoring, volunteering, designing clothes, interior designing, building something, remodeling, your contribution to a project at work, research, learning something new, time with the Divine—the sky's the limit! There's no right or wrong answer.

❖ Once you've found what it is, be sure you get enough of it on a daily or weekly basis, if possible. You might even consider changing jobs or picking up a second job or volunteering. Consider the following:
  • *What lights you up?*
  • *What energizes you?*
  • *What drains you?*
  • *Where's the void in your life?*
  • *What's missing?*

It's never too late to do what you love and serve your purpose!

Eliminate the Need for Willpower

Once you begin your spiritual journey, seeing who you really are and what you are meant for, your beliefs and values start to shift toward that which supports your purpose and authenticity. It makes you think twice about all that you strive for and seek to obtain. (This is something I'm still working on every day!) You start considering what you *really* want and making decisions to support that desire. It all starts to clearly align, so willpower isn't even necessary. You just naturally start to move and eat in ways that support who you are and that better enable you to fill your purpose and be fulfilled.

Use Gratitude to Give You Perspective and Energy!

There will be times when we stray from what we know to be best. There's nothing like gratitude to keep us in check. It humbles us and allows us to be more satisfied with less. It has a way of bringing out the best in every person and situation. Stephen Grable, MD, of Complementary Care Center in Jacksonville, Florida, suggests you make it a part of your daily practice to express gratitude in some way. He says that if you can be grateful for hardships, it completely changes your outlook and allows you to experience more joy and positive energy in your life. He refers to the "law of attraction" as a reminder that what we focus on is what we bring into our lives. He says, "Quantum physicists have proven that our emotions and thoughts are energy. In other words, you're affecting your physical body with your emotions and thoughts."[71]

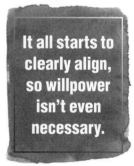

It all starts to clearly align, so willpower isn't even necessary.

The apostle Paul, whose life was characterized by hardship and suffering, conveys the same essential message in one of his letters: "Summing it all up, friends, I'd say you'll do best by filling your minds and meditating on things true, noble, reputable, authentic, compelling, gracious—the best, not the worst; the beautiful, not the ugly; things to praise, not things to curse" (Philippians 4:8).[72]

---

71   Dr. Stephen Grable, interview with author on August 3, 2017.

72   Philippians 4:8, The Message Bible.

In his book *The Art of Stopping Time*, Pedram Shojai, OMD, says, "Gratitude is good medicine and is always time well spent. It helps relieve stress and build positive energy, and it gives us great perspective on life."[73]

Unlock the Key to Weight Loss

When you find pleasure in the simple things and frequently participate in activities and work that you enjoy, you're *naturally* **happy, free, more creative and loving**. You can see how you fill a unique purpose in this world, deriving satisfaction from that role, instead of turning to food to fulfill an unmet longing.

When you realize how **unique you are**, ==>
==> you can really **love yourself**, ==>
==> which is to **take care of yourself** ==>
==> so you can **serve your purpose**.

> You can see how you fill a unique purpose in this world, deriving satisfaction from that role, instead of turning to food to fulfill an unmet longing.

Did you get that? Did you grasp how those steps flow? If you missed it, you just might be missing the whole point and find yourself backtracking on your health journey. If you don't really understand and love yourself, you're going to do things that might feel good temporarily but you know will harm you in the long run and put you even further away from reaching your goals. On the other hand, when you know, love, and accept yourself, understanding that you're here to serve a greater purpose, your decisions take on a whole

---

73   Pedram Shojai, OMD, *The Art of Stopping Time* (New York: Rodale, 2017), 3.

new perspective. It becomes so much easier to walk away from the junk food, not because you *can't* have it, but because you know how it will make you feel and how it will affect your health, thus preventing you from being the best version of yourself that you were meant to be. So the next time you go to reach for food that is void of nutrients and serves you no purpose, ask yourself what you *really* want. What will fill that longing, that void in your soul? **What will make you smile on the inside?**

Define Your *Why*

Now that we've explored your purpose and ways to fill your spirit and soul, I want you to think about a very meaningful exercise that could make the difference in achieving and not achieving your health goals. In the last chapter, I introduced you to the holistic elements of health—mind, body, and spirit. But beyond that, on a more personal level, **what does health mean to *you*?** Most people would say it's related to the state of being free from illness or injury, a person's mental or physical condition, well-being, fitness, good condition, vigor, strength, good shape, wellness. Maybe a better way to phrase the last question is, ***Why* do you want to be healthy?** For me, being healthy meant I didn't have to wonder if I would wake up feeling bad every morning. It meant I could get through the day without the distraction of having to refuel my "dead batteries" every afternoon. It meant I wouldn't have to depend on medication to sustain me, no more regular doctor's visits, that I could be stronger for my family instead of

> **Your WHY is the first step to success and has the power to always keep you on track as you visit it and revisit it throughout your health journey.**

always depending on someone else to get things done. It also meant I wouldn't be consumed and tormented by every piece of food I put in my mouth, that I could just naturally eat what I know supports me in feeling my best! It meant I could feel good putting on my favorite pair of jeans and not having to stand in my closet for hours trying to find something that fits. It also meant I'd have the confidence to wear cute summer clothes and be ready for the next big event (vacation, someone's wedding, class reunion, etc.) without panicking and having to jump on a fast-results diet. Ultimately, *my* why is so I can fulfill my purpose of helping others feel and look *their* best too!

So what about you? Now it's your turn to figure out your why. Love yourself enough to figure out how your life could be different, how it could be so much better if you had your optimal health back. Your WHY is the first step to success and has the power to always keep you on track as you visit it and revisit it throughout your health journey. Keep in mind that your why will more than likely change throughout your lifetime as life takes you on different journeys at different stages. That's why it's good to build a strong support system and be proactive and mindful by reassessing your why from time to time.

Receive a free step-by-step guide to helping you explore and define YOUR WHY to help you kick-start your success by going to www.leahcampian.com/your-why.

Scan this QR code to receive your FREE step-by-step guide to helping you explore and define YOUR WHY! (Valued at $25)

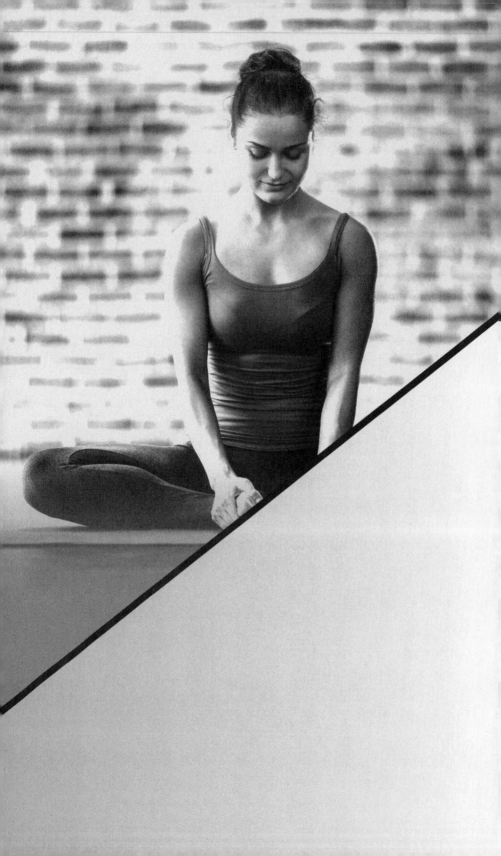

Chapter 8

What Doesn't Work:
A Restricted Mindset

"As a man thinks in his heart, so is he."[74]

—Proverbs 23:7

"It's not what happens to you, but how you respond to it that matters."

—Epictetus

---

74   Proverbs 23:7, The Holy Bible (Modern English Version).

*"To thrive is to manage your health
without being managed by it."*[75]

—Dr. Alan Christianson

*"Instead of trying to break a habit, think
about transforming a habit."*[76]

—Alexandra Jamieson

*"Learning to develop gentle and tender thoughts first
toward yourself, then toward others, goes a long way."*[77]

—Dori Thomsen, Owner and Instructor at Soluna Yoga & Spa

The previous chapter covers our spiritual dimension. Now let's take a closer look at our mind and its impact on our health. I want to show you the psychology behind making lifestyle changes that stick.

God gave us the sense we need to protect ourselves and thrive—for example, we have enough sense to find shelter in a storm or to escape a fire. Those reactions are innate and would be foolish to ignore. Yet it's just as foolish to ignore the dangers of certain behaviors, harmful substances, or our body's negative reactions to certain foods,

---

75   Christianson, 172.

76   Jamieson, 46.

77   Dori Thomsen, interview with author on June 26, 2017.

wouldn't you agree? To do that is like standing out in the middle of a tornado, just hoping and praying we don't get swept away or hit by flying debris!

When I hear people saying that certain foods hurt them when eaten yet they continue consuming them, knowing they're doing harm to themselves, I can't help but stand back in astonishment. How can these behaviors be justified? Why would someone continue harming themselves? Well, it's a lot like alcoholism or smoking. There must be some other benefit to continuing that behavior. And in that person's mind, the temporary gain outweighs the potential losses if the habit ends. It's certainly understandable that these addictions can be hard to break, and there are also many other factors like convenience and ignorance when it comes to finding alternatives, but that's a big part of my purpose for writing this book—I know it's hard, but what's hard at first becomes easier, and caring goes a very long way. When you're interested in becoming a better person, you'll want to look into what it takes to achieve that goal and will begin trying new things, propelled by your excitement for positive change! However, you've got to realize early on that it won't always be easy to stay the course, and that you'll want to throw in the towel when you've had enough. That's where I come in to help you identify and overcome those destructive behaviors and to keep pushing through, despite your feelings. Rick Stollmeyer, CEO of MINDBODY, says, "Modern life is making healthy living harder." That is certainly true and something we can't ignore, but what are you going to do about it? I've already made my decision, but I can't make yours for you. Are you going to let someone else or something else control your

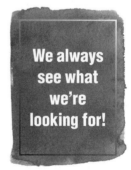

We always see what we're looking for!

outcome, or are you going to define your own destiny? Rick also says, "You've got to win the battle inside your head before seeing change in the body."[78]

Mind over Matter

If we really understood the power of the mind, we could do anything! Often the difference between successful and unsuccessful people, champions and the mediocre, is the mind. The successful see what they *can* do and don't allow what they *can't* do into their heads, whereas the mediocre pay too much attention to the negative chatter in their minds. You see, our minds have not been endowed with intrinsic objectivity. We see *everything* through our mind's eye. It's called *perspective*. Thoughts come and go like clouds. It's the thoughts we choose to entertain and give attention to that can hold us back or move us forward. Remember this: Thoughts become words, words become behaviors, and behaviors become actions and habits. It's that simple! **So by changing your *outlook*, you can change your life.** What a difference perspective can make! The victim sees something that has happened *to* them, whereas the opportunist sees that the same thing has happened *for* them. When you see that something has happened *for* you, it is eye-opening! You can do something about it. Act on it. It's the same situation, but now there are so many more possibilities. You're not stuck. So start looking for what you *want* because we always see what we're looking for! I love how Lysa Terkeurst puts it: "What if this whole journey of getting healthy could be more about what we're in the process of gaining than what

> In order to experience lasting change, you'll need to understand the reasons behind your patterns.

---

78   Rick Stollmeyer, interview with author on July 21, 2017.

we're losing?"[79] "Focusing only on what we're giving up will make us feel constantly deprived. And deprivation leads to desperation, frustration, and failure.... See the gains as more valuable than the losses."[80]

Let Go of the Past

No one but *you* decides the power you give to the past. This is a big obstacle for some people making progress that sticks when trying to improve and maintain their health. While it can be productive to visit our past experiences in order to learn and understand our present emotions and behaviors, it's important to *let those experiences go.* A coach is especially skilled at helping you see things from a different perspective in order for you to accept your story, experience those feelings, and use the power of those past experiences to *unleash your potential* in the present, going forward. Of course, there are times when a therapist needs to get involved, but most of us can deal with our past and move on, with just a little willingness and guidance. Understanding our connection with past experiences and present feelings and behaviors allows us insight into some of our triggers. In order to experience lasting change, you'll need to understand the reasons behind your patterns. Sometimes it's just a matter of nostalgia, where a certain time of year, smell, place, reminds us of a past experience that was tied to foods we've decided aren't the best choices for us now. It's good to find healthy replacements, but sometimes, every now and then, it's also good to have what you're craving.

> We must understand our own bent to understand the message that will resonate with us individually.

---

79   Terkeurst, 179.
80   Terkeurst, 181.

I find that the longer I go without the junk, when I do give in and have it, it usually makes me sick or doesn't taste as good as I thought it would or doesn't give me what I was looking for, and that ends up being the end of that escapade!

Streamline Decisions Based on Your Personality

We've all heard the phrase "you are your own worst enemy." I can understand how it can happen. Take, for example, a type A personality, someone who might have OCD or is overly controlling. This person does not need to tell themselves to get off the couch and go for a run. In fact, it might do them good to take a break, stop running marathons, and instead get involved in a yoga class. On the other hand, a laid-back, indecisive personality might need a nudge to get moving, or a scheduled routine to keep them on track. We must understand our own bent to understand the message that will resonate with us individually. Because we're creatures of habit, it's helpful to recognize our own tendencies and triggers, and by doing so, we can **automate our decisions** and change our environment to promote new behaviors. The idea of automation involves making a decision in support of our goals, then putting a plan in place to achieve those goals—without waver, without question—because it is something that has become part of our mindset, our routine, a habit, and is now second nature to us. For example, if I decided that I will practice yoga every other morning, I will set my yoga clothes out the night prior, set the alarm early enough to fit in that exercise, saying to myself, "I practice yoga every other day," as if it is *a fact* already. If I want to eat healthy, I will pack healthy lunches for myself either on the weekends or the evenings before I work, to ensure that I **leave nothing to happenstance**. After a while, these things become a part of me, without question.

Understand Food's Influence on Your Mind

Another important part of making your transformation permanent is to learn how your brain works. Why is it that when I say I want to lose weight and know that eating pizza will keep me from achieving that goal, I still choose to eat the pizza? While there could be many reasons, as we've seen throughout the book thus far, the following culprits can have a great impact on our choices. Understanding them and how to find solutions to work around them will be **KEY in unlocking your struggles with maintaining healthy habits**. Once you become aware of them and learn to recognize them, you'll understand that it's not really your fault and that no amount of willpower or self-discipline can combat the stronghold they have on your mind, behaviors, and actions. If you're a child of the '80s and '90s or older, you might remember the TV commercial "Your brain on drugs..." Well, let's talk about your *brain on food* or so-called food!

1. **Emotional eating** is a big driver of bad decisions, as it results in destructive patterns that keep us from moving forward. We crave some foods due to mental conditioning; that is, our minds have conditioned us to feel certain emotions when we think of, see, smell, or eat some foods because those foods are tied to certain life events. That is our mind's way of satisfying a need, sometimes not even evoking a good emotion; yet it is a familiar one, which can bring a certain level of comfort. We do sometimes eat when we aren't hungry due to positive emotions, and we also use food and the activity of eating to turn off or avoid certain emotions that cause pain or that we don't feel comfortable with experiencing or don't want to deal with.

How negative emotions can drive us to eat:

- ❖ When we're **angry**, we often go for something *crunchy*.
- ❖ When we're **lonely**, food becomes our *companion*.
- ❖ When we've been **hurt**, we like something *sweet* or *smooth and creamy* to comfort us.
- ❖ When we're **tired or exhausted**, we go for *sugar* or *caffeine* to energize us.
- ❖ When we're **wired** and need to relax, we go for *alcohol* or *stuff ourselves* so we're too tired to do anything else and must rest.
- ❖ Even **guilt and shame** can push us to eat as a way of **stuffing those feelings back inside** instead of dealing with them.

A coach can help you discover different ways to celebrate and express positive emotions as alternatives to eating unnecessarily. On the other hand, if you're overeating foods that don't support your health due to negative emotions or feelings, you'll need to learn to deal with those emotions in a different way. At the end of this chapter, I'll teach you a couple of useful techniques you can try out to change the way you respond to your triggers.

2. **Cravings** become a constant struggle for most of us, often winning the battle we wage from within, no matter how strong our willpower. Cravings can be prompted for various reasons, but almost always due to an imbalance.

- ❖ Many diets are very restrictive and don't promote balanced nutrition, which has an effect on our minds. We can crave certain foods because of a chemical imbalance that is produced when we lack certain nutrients.

- Most of the time, cravings are signaling to the body that it's missing out on something unrelated to food. Even something as simple as a lack of sleep can cause cravings. Robb Wolf, in his book *Wired to Eat*, explains, "Not only do we tend to crave highly processed foods when sleep deprived, but we also tend to have less willpower to resist these foods."[81] Wondering how much sleep you need? Dr. Sara Gottfried cites studies that show only 3% to 4% of the population has the ability to function well on little sleep.[82] Most people need seven to eight and a half hours of sleep every day.

- Focus on your gaps with the primary foods, identified in Chapter 6, to discover how you might be able to satisfy those cravings for something more in your life.

- The book *Women, Food, and Desire* by Alexandra Jamieson is a great resource for better understanding cravings and healthy alternatives to satisfying them. "When we start building in more pleasure, whether emotional, physical, or even imagined, cravings for food lose their power over us."[83]

> **Cravings can be prompted for various reasons, but almost always due to an imbalance.**

- This is another hot topic with practical tips in my Ditch the Diet Program or any private coaching session with clients! To learn more about these services, go to www.leahcampian.com/ditch-the-diet-program.

---

81 Wolf, 114.

82 Gottfried, *The Hormone Cure*.

83 Jamieson, 95.

3. **Food addictions** are also good at derailing us from our intentions. Even the most self-disciplined among us can struggle with food addiction. Addiction is when you keep doing something in the face of mounting consequences. Just like the other triggers that play games with our minds, food addictions are a *biological* response.

  ❖ The **chemicals** in processed foods keep us addicted and coming back for more, even when we know we might not feel so great after making that food choice. We just can't help it—we're addicted! Food scientists are challenged by mega food companies to make food that consumers will want more of in order to increase the company's sales. The books *Pandora's Lunchbox*[84] by Melanie Warner and *Salt Sugar Fat*[85] by Michael Moss have a lot more on our processed food systems.

  ❖ **Sugar (see Chapter 4) and gluten** are good for wreaking this same havoc!

    Sugar lights up the same part of the brain that is activated by cocaine consumption. Not only does it have that effect on the brain, which creates a very strong addiction, but also, as discussed, in Chapter 4, it causes issues with our blood sugar levels and gut, requiring constant consumption to get our fix, like a steady drip of drugs from an IV bag. When we eat too much sugar, our guts also become out of balance, with bad bacteria or yeast taking over the good bacteria and causing cravings. The yeast lives off sugar and convinces you to keep feeding it,

---

84 Warner, *Pandora's Lunchbox.*

85 Michael Moss, *Salt Sugar Fat: How the Food Giants Hooked Us* (New York: Random House, 2013).

thus making you an addict! Innately, we know that sugar of any kind will give us energy, so it's the body's natural way of maintaining our energy levels, especially for those of us whose energy stores are quickly depleted by all the demands and high-stress situations we put on ourselves. We just need to keep in mind all that we learned about sugar in Chapter 4, giving ourselves the better-quality options, and more importantly, trying alternatives to maintaining our energy levels.

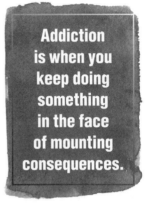

Addiction is when you keep doing something in the face of mounting consequences.

Gluten has an *opiate-like effect* on the brain, working like a drug as well. Not only does it cause gut issues and blood-sugar imbalances, but it is addicting, so the more we eat, the more we want, making it hard to quit. Dr. Tom O'Bryan is a great resource for all things gluten.[86] He says that while the media and many celebrities have made gluten-free diets a fad, there's no fad to the science: The fact is that no human has the digestive enzymes to fully digest wheat proteins into individual amino acids, which would be necessary for proper digestion of proteins. While we may have a tolerance to these minor toxins initially, at some point or another, we'll cross a line of tolerance and develop an intolerance that can lead to inflammation caused by antibodies circulating through our bloodstream.

---

86   Tom O'Bryan, DC, CCN, DACBN, *The Autoimmune Fix: How to Stop the Hidden Autoimmune Damage That Keeps You Sick, Fat, and Tired Before It Turns into Disease* (New York: Rodale, 2016).

These antibodies are so dangerous because of their ability to mimic various molecules in our body, making us vulnerable to a plethora of issues.[87]

"From autism to infertility, from the tummy to the brain, from the heart to the joints, from gallstones to tears in the protective 'cheesecloth' of the brain called the Blood-Brain-Barrier (emphasis mine), there is no system of the body that is immune to disease from problems in the gut."[88]

If the health of our brain is in our gut, we'd better start focusing on that first! In the same paper, Dr. O'Bryan gets more specific in reactions to gluten: "From Inflammatory Bowel Disease (Ulcerative Colitis and Crohn's Disease), to numerous autoimmune diseases (Rheumatoid Arthritis, Psoriasis, Type 1 Diabetes, Spondylitis, etc.), from Gluten Sensitivity and Celiac disease, to Food Allergies, from Neurological conditions (Autism Spectrum Disorder, Depression, Anxiety, ADHD, Guillain-Barré Syndrome, etc.)... the list goes on and on of the symptoms that may be triggered by Intestinal Permeability. This is why Intestinal Permeability has been called 'The Gateway to Autoimmunity.'" If everything hinges on our gut health, it would behoove us to learn all we can to take precious care of it. With modern science, we're fortunate to have the ability to

It's up to *you* to learn the truth and make the necessary changes to reclaim your health.

---

87   Dr. Tom O'Bryan, interview with author on October 27, 2017.

88   www.theDr.com, accessed January 22, 2018, www.thedr.com/all-about-gluten/articles/intestinal-problems-and-whole-body-symptoms-gut-101-the-effect-of-foods-as-written-for-autism-one/.

pinpoint the root cause of many of our issues and make changes to help us beyond our issues instead of continuing down a path of hindering ourselves from being well. This is a big topic worth researching more to learn how you could be impacted and what to do about it. A few excellent resources are the books *The Autoimmune Fix* by Tom O'Bryan, DC, CCN, DACBN[89]; *Wheat Belly* by William Davis, MD[90]; and *Grain Brain* by David Perlmutter, MD.[91]

Most of the junk in our diets today is loaded with sugar and gluten, both causing a quick rise in blood sugar levels, then a sudden crash, leaving us craving more, just like drug addicts. Isn't it interesting that so many addicting drugs are illegal, and even tobacco and alcohol are illegal for the underage; but these addicting food substances that are destroying our health and causing an epidemic of diabetes, obesity, heart disease, digestive issues, behavioral disorders, and autoimmune diseases are not just allowed but *heavily pushed* in our society, especially to the youngest, most susceptible individuals? This is yet another reminder that you can't outsource your health! It's up to *you* to learn the truth and make the necessary changes to reclaim your health.

Learn to get comfortable with being uncomfortable. While we don't want to depend on willpower or self-control alone, we certainly have to use them, especially while we learn how to become less reliant on them. Willpower and self-control are necessary when we're faced with uncomfortable situations, but what if we could learn to be okay with the discomfort? That's one of the first things I learned in yoga class.

---

89   O'Bryan, *The Autoimmune Fix.*

90   William Davis, MD, *Wheat Belly: Lose the Wheat, Lose the Weight, and Find Your Path Back to Health* (New York: Rodale, 2011).

91   David Perlmutter, MD with Loberg, Kristin. *Grain Brain: The Surprising Truth About Wheat, Carbs, and Sugar – Your Brain's Silent Killers* (New York: Hachette Book Group, 2013).

Discomfort is a sign of change. Think about children and their physical growing pains. A teething baby cries from pain, and as much as you hate to see them suffer, you would never stop the process, because you know it would stop their growth and development. Why would we do the same thing to ourselves? I like to think of discomfort as a rite of passage for moving to the next level. When I was a freshman in high school, my sister went off to college, and I was looked to as the one to replace her playing the piano for a choir. I remember her teaching me the songs and how hard it was for me to stretch into that role. Not only did it entail new techniques I hadn't learned before, but also I was trying to fill the shoes of an amazing pianist who could easily play by ear and had won many awards for her skills. I remember thinking I could never do it, and I'd be so nervous every week as I went to play. Looking back, I am so grateful for that opportunity of being "pushed" into those uncomfortable situations. I can honestly attribute my abilities as an advanced pianist today to that and other similar situations. Had I quit or refused to accept those challenges, just think—I might not be as successful as I am today!

It can actually be comforting to be content with discomfort, yet we often mistakenly associate discomfort with something being wrong, which is not always the case.

"People who truly thrive realize that life offers many opportunities in which being willing to take on temporary discomfort means greater happiness later."[92]

—Dr. Alan Christianson

---

92   Christianson, 171.

Have you ever heard the saying "The way you do one thing is the way you do everything"? I see it every day in my own life, as well as the life of those around me and my clients. For example, once I learned to get uncomfortable in yoga class and just sit with it, it strengthened me in other ways. I gained calmness about myself, an understanding that I am stronger than I gave myself credit for, a peace with just being without doing, and the increased ability to delay gratification, to say no to my immediate desire, for greater gain at some future time. If you can stand there, with your body shaking, sweat dripping down every part of your body, itching to scratch, dying to move, you'll reap the benefit of a deeper stretch next time, the next, and the next, until you can achieve what you once thought was impossible, and have a new body to show for it! The same is true in every area of our lives, so do yourself a big favor and learn to get comfortable with being uncomfortable.

> **I like to think of discomfort as a rite of passage for moving to the next level.**

See How Your Fear Can Open Many Doors

Hey, I've got some good news for you: *Fear* doesn't mean *failure*. It's completely natural to experience fear. I think the biggest fear for most people is *the unknown*. People also greatly fear *change* because they might be uncomfortable and have to go through unfamiliar situations. There's something comforting about familiarity and knowing, even if you *know* it's not working and are *familiar* with all the negative impacts. While those feelings are illogical, they bring comfort through familiarity. Don't worry; you're not alone. What determines whether you'll be successful or not is how you learn to deal with your fear. There are three steps that allow you to start turning your fear into courage:

1. **Embrace it.** Begin to accept the way you're feeling. Just sit with it, and fully experience those emotions, even if it makes you uncomfortable. Believe me, no one is comfortable with facing their fears.

2. **Let it teach you.** Once you've embraced the fear, what can you learn from it? Is it revealing something about you? Do your past experiences have something to do with it? Determine the worst-case scenario, and answer this question: "So what?" "If *abc*... so what?"

3. **Don't let it hold you back.** We're really good at imagining the worst possible outcome, but why not give more attention to the *best*-case scenario? Follow that best-case scenario. Now you're ready to take action because the fear has taught you something about yourself and different possibilities and outcomes that you might not have been open to considering before.

Learn to make this sequence automatic. When I'm paralyzed with fear, I use it as my catalyst to ACT, MOVE, and *DO IT*! Let me be vulnerable for a moment. I had to face this when writing and finishing this book. Here's where you have to fight your instinct to hide or run away and instead seize the opportunity to jump right on it and tackle that fear. A health coach can guide you through these steps, as it can be a difficult experience on your own, especially at first try. One thing I learned from one of my coaches is that most decisions aren't final and that it's more about our reactions to the consequences of our choices than it is about the consequences themselves. That's really what life is

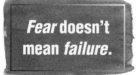

Fear doesn't mean failure.

all about—how we choose to *react* to circumstances. We're human, we're going to make mistakes, but there's power in acknowledging that those choices aren't final.

There's always something more. There's always another series of choices that can change our path and direction. By choosing to focus on the positive rather than the negative, you're freeing yourself from restraints your mind has put on you. While our instincts can protect us, some of us get hung up on the small chance that something bad might happen and never live life to its fullest. Learn to focus instead on the big chance that awesome things will happen for you. And when the bad things happen, think about how they happened *for* you rather than *to* you.

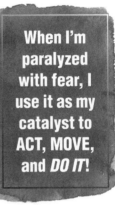

When I'm paralyzed with fear, I use it as my catalyst to ACT, MOVE, and *DO IT*!

How Do You Make the Best Choices?

"Often, when people are in situations in which they cannot meet their ideal standards, they abandon all standards."[93]

—Dr. Alan Christianson

To keep you on track throughout your health journey, it will be important for you to learn how to make good decisions based on your set goals by analyzing the reasons behind your desires. This is a fundamental part of my coaching sessions with clients and also a part of the Ditch the Diet Program. Here I've provided a tool to help you move quickly through the decision-making process. Become familiar with this list of pivotal questions, then pause in that moment and ask yourself one or more of them:

---

93   Christianson, 172.

* Why do I *want* this?
* How does it *serve* me or my purpose?
* Is it *worthy* of me?
* How do I feel right now, and what am I *hoping to feel* from this experience?

So here you are, faced with a box of donuts a coworker has brought into the office. As you go through that last series of questions, it will help you understand:

* The junk that's been set before you is **not, in fact, worthy of you** at all.
* **Your value cannot be measured.** That donut is worth a dime, while the true cost to you could be destruction (health issues, guilt and shame, lack of confidence, determent from meeting your weight loss goals, etc.). When comparing her chips and chocolate to her courage, Lysa Terkeurst says, "My courage is so much more valuable and beautiful and empowering and lasting."[94]
* The only **purpose it may serve** is to give you immediate energy and maybe even some form of comfort, to relieve stress and tension.
* So maybe that's **why you really want it**. Right now you feel sluggish and tired, stressed and tense, so this worthless junk will have some power over you, to comfort you, as it may have in the past.

Those questions are pivotal because they hold the power to pivot you into the right direction—away from the danger you may be facing. Once you honestly answer those questions, you're **empowered to make better decisions**, to meet your needs in other ways that are better aligned with who you are, what you want, and thus your goals. Deborah Rozman, co-CEO of HeartMath and co-author of the

---

94   Terkeurst, 181.

book *Stopping Emotional Eating*,[95] says that "maintaining our health is hard because we struggle to manage our emotions. Things like overwhelming stress and a lack of support can cause behavioral issues and breakdowns, where we just get 'stuck in our heads,' controlled by our emotions. It becomes a fight between the heart and mind." She suggests we qualify our perceptions and actions through our heart. That's what she calls "heart-based living." "This is done by pausing and focusing on your heart, which sends a different message to your brain to change your perception of a situation. Listening to your heart's intuitive intelligence can guide you to make better choices that are different from your emotional desires or mental concerns."[96] I like how she categorizes the way we decide:

- The mind says, "I can't."
- The emotions say, "I really want xyz."
- But the heart is truer to what the body needs.

A health coach can help you identify replacements and better choices, depending on your individuality. This is where the one-size-fits-all approach is simply not going to function. Having a coach is like having a sounding board. Working closely with someone who learns more about your unique personality and needs is a great way to apply what might work best for you!

---

95   Deborah Rozman and Doc Childre. *Stopping Emotional Eating: Heartmath Stress and Weight Management Program* (Cardiff: Waterfront Digital Press, 2017).

96   Deborah Rozman, interview with author on July 13, 2017.

"It's ironic, isn't it? Knowing that when we can just stop and do nothing—even for a brief moment— that's when we actually regain control."[97]

—Alexandra Jamieson

You Eat What You Are

That's right. I didn't get it backwards. We've all heard the saying "You are what you eat," and in some ways that's true, but we also eat based on the way we see ourselves. When exhausted, confused, frustrated, unsatisfied, what do you eat? I know what I want to go for! Donuts, fries, pizza, ice cream, and the list goes on—right? You just want to sit on the couch and engage in mindless activities, like checking social media, playing video games or watching TV, something to numb the pain, fill the boredom, or to distract yourself from thinking about your situation so you won't have to deal with it. You even start using laughter as a crutch to hide your true feelings. You start seeing the bad in everyone else so you don't feel so bad about yourself. You treat them the way you feel about yourself, with no respect. In psychology, it's referred to as *projection*. You project your feelings about yourself onto others. If you're able to relate to any of the examples, don't feel bad. These behaviors are **subconscious**, just *automatic reactions* to our feelings. So how do you change them? When you know your purpose and your value, you make decisions to support who you are. If **you are** life and energy, that's what you eat! Whole foods have life and energy from the sun and earth, unlike the processed foods made to last on the shelf for months. You start moving in a vibrant way as an expression of

---

97   Jamieson, 95.

that life and energy. *It's a cycle that keeps feeding itself, one behavior after another.* Laughter comes from the joy **deep down inside** and is **reflected** on your face as it shines, and in the way you see and treat others—with respect, without judgment, seeing them for *their* **true value** because you were able to first see yourself for your true value. I remember when this shift started taking place within me. What a liberating transformation! Suddenly, food choices weren't a struggle anymore. I knew exactly what I was meant for and what I needed to eat to support that meaning. I like how Bill Di Stanisloa of Farm Life Foundation puts it so simply: "The food must follow the thought. When the thought follows the food, it ends in disease."[98]

Think about the high school wrestling champ or the Olympic swimmer. They have the freedom to eat whatever they want, to do whatever they want, but because of their talent, they have a purpose to fulfill. Maybe it's just breaking a personal record, maybe it's winning the next tournament, or maybe it's taking gold home for their country. Either way, they understand that while they have the freedom to choose, they maintain discipline because they know it will strengthen them to meet their objective. In other words, just because they *can* doesn't mean they *should*. Whether you're the CEO of an organization that needs your critical thinking skills or the teacher of a fifth-grade class of students who need your energy and passion, your daily decisions begin to shift when you see *yourself* in a different light. Think about how wonderful this world could be if we all lived up to our own potential. It gives me goose bumps to imagine it!

> When you know your purpose and your value, you make decisions to support who you are.

---

98 Bill Di Stanisloa, interview with author on June 27, 2017.

Give Yourself a Break

Boy that sounds nice, huh? The truth is that you *will* mess up and make mistakes. Instead of beating yourself up for it, *learn* from those mistakes. Don't give yourself permission to have a bad day based on one poor decision, and don't give yourself permission to have a bad week based on one day of poor decisions—no more "I'll start fresh on Monday" business! Doesn't that pattern seem

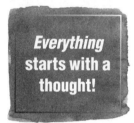

Everything starts with a thought!

familiar? It's the pattern of those of us who have struggled to make change permanent in our lives. A great way to get out of this pattern is by putting the "rules of the game" on paper. For example:

- ❖ If I mess up, I will not use that as an excuse to continue in a downward spiral.
- ❖ I will explore why I made the mistake to help myself not go down that path again.
- ❖ Example exploration: When I feel tired, my body naturally looks for something that will energize it, so I reach for something sweet for immediate energy. But then I feel like crap after I eat it and still want more a couple of hours later.
- ❖ Lesson learned:
  - • Stay rested as much as possible.
  - • Move my body regularly for natural energy.
  - • Stay prepared with healthy snacks that will boost my energy.
  - • Eat a regular diet of organic whole foods, full of the Earth's energy.
  - • Stop and breathe, inhaling energy-enhancing aromas for a couple of minutes in that moment to increase my energy levels.

Write your own story, and improve it each time you write! **There's something powerful about putting your thoughts on paper**, but if that's too much for you, just start by *changing the story you tell yourself.* What you tell yourself, over and over again, you believe, and those beliefs form the values by which you live. (Remember the cycle from Chapter 2?) *Everything* starts with a thought! I like the perspective author Michael Neill puts on a "train of thoughts." We choose to entertain a series of thoughts by getting on that "train" of thoughts leading us in a certain direction that ultimately leads to a specific destination. But in choosing to get off the train of negativity, for example, by not entertaining those thoughts, we don't get where that train was heading. We can instead choose to board another train that will take us to the destination where we really want to end up.[99] When you get off track, go back to your system. What message are you feeding yourself? Are you believing truths or lies?

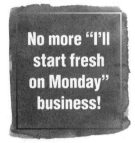

No more "I'll start fresh on Monday" business!

Affirm the Actions That Will Help You Reach Your Goals

To affirm, state as a fact, declare one's support for, uphold or defend, offer (someone) emotional support or encouragement (definitions from Merriam-Webster and Dictionary.com). This is a wonderful technique that is quite simple but takes some time to master. The idea is to take the things that you don't necessarily enjoy doing or that aren't easy for you but that you know will help you reach your health goals and state them as facts about yourself. For example:

---

99   Michael Neill, *Supercoach: 10 Secrets to Transform Anyone's Life* (New York: Hay House Inc., 2009), 112.

- ❖ I wake up 10 minutes early to meditate so I'll have a balanced day.
- ❖ I eat vegetables for the energy they give me.
- ❖ I eat mindfully to enjoy my food and nourish my body fully.
- ❖ I plan my meals a week in advance so I can stay on track and feel great.
- ❖ I go to yoga class every Tuesday and Thursday.

The benefit of such statements is that even though you may not yet "believe" them, you're feeding your mind with what you want to happen. And when repeated enough, you begin to believe what you've been saying. If you were to begin doing something different, your mind might say, "Hey, wait! I don't eat junk. I eat food that gives me the Earth's energy," or "Oh yeah, tomorrow's Tuesday, so I'd better get my gym bag ready for yoga class after work."

Now take a look at the definition with me. Not only are you making factual statements, but also you're "supporting, upholding, defending" and providing emotional support and encouragement to yourself! That seems pretty powerful to me for something so simple and totally FREE! Try it on by putting these statements in writing and carrying them around with you so when you see them, you say them over and over again. You'll need to do this for about a month to really benefit. Once you believe enough to take consistent action and see the magic transforming your behaviors and turning them into good habits, you'll see that you no longer need the written statements, and you'll be ready to take on newer and bigger affirmations!

> **Positive thoughts can take our minds where we eventually want to be.**

Tap into Your Mind as a Power Source

❖ **Visualization** is a very powerful technique used by many to achieve their goals. Just as negative thoughts and images can plague our minds, positive thoughts can take our minds where we eventually want to be. You can start with a guided visualization offered by many experts in just about any area of interest. While listening to a guided form gives you the idea of how it's done, you'll want to discover this method on your own. The simplest way is to imagine what you would look like if you met your goal weight. What would you be wearing? Where would you be? What would you be doing? How would you feel? You get the idea. It's important to revisit these visualizations over and over. They'll become an integral part of your new lifestyle, changing the way you *do* things because of the way you've *seen* things in your visualizations.

> It's as if the story in your head became reality, helping you to see it as though it were already part of your habits.

❖ **Cognitive behavioral therapy** is another technique used to change behaviors and habits. It's similar to visualization, yet different because you revisit an event or situation where you didn't act in a way that supports your ideals, goals, best interests, etc. And by revisiting, I mean, you go back to the place, the sounds, the scenery, the smells, what you were wearing, how you felt in that moment, and just before making the wrong decision... that's where your mind changes the story. So instead of pulling into the fast-food drive-thru, you do something else like get a cup of soup and a wrap from a health food store, or go home and cook something delicious, or take a walk in the park. You get the idea. The benefit in changing your story in your mind is that the next time you're faced with the same choice, you behave according to the ideal that you painted in your head. It's as if the story in your head became reality, helping you to see it as though it were already part of your habits.

> **Happiness won't come where worry exists.**

While there are many other tools and techniques, those are two of my favorites, as they're very simple and powerful, and can be done anywhere, anytime. Give them a try sometime. I think you'll be pleasantly surprised with the results!

This chapter was, by far, my favorite to write and read. It's full of nuggets of truth and wisdom, with practical applications. I hope you'll revisit it as often as you need. In closing this chapter, I want to point out that a healthy lifestyle has no room for worry. Remember the song "Don't worry, be happy"? Keep in mind that it has two parts to it. Happiness won't come where worry exists. That's the power your mind holds. Don't fuel it with worry. Instead, choose to be happy.

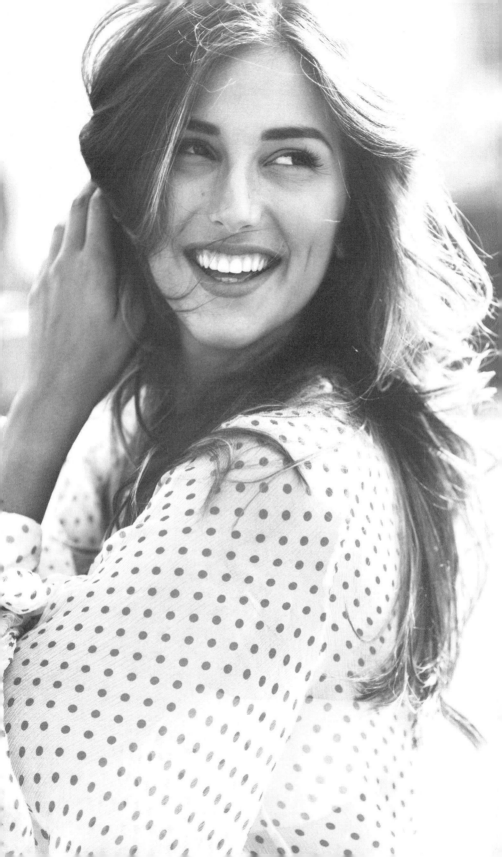

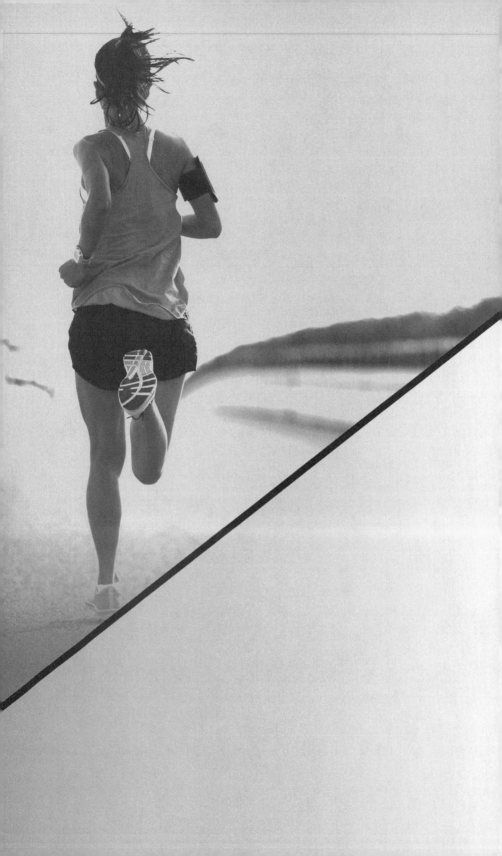

What Doesn't Work:
A Short-Term Outlook

"It's your road, and yours alone. Others may walk it with you, but no one can walk it for you."

—Jalaluddin Rumi

"Don't try to do everything at once. Build on it. Learn to love your vegetables."[100]

—Justine Kelly, Sun Basket Chef

---

100   Justine Kelly, interview with author on June 29, 2017.

> *"Don't do something for two weeks if you don't see yourself doing it in two years."*[101]

—Lisa Powell, MS, RDN, Nutrition Director at Canyon Ranch

With temporary goals in mind, my focus was always on the short term—fitting into a dress for a friend's wedding, looking good in my bikini on my next cruise, finishing a long race, etc. While there isn't necessarily anything wrong with those goals, they skew your mentality of what's *most* important in life. It's really about the journey, not one or even many destinations. Sometimes those short-term goals can prevent us from putting enough focus on what it takes to maintain our health so we can enjoy this journey and make it last even longer!

Expert Advice

Pedram Shojai, author of *The Urban Monk*, says that for permanent transformation to take place, "You have to understand that your health, vitality, energy, time, and money are all part of the same force. To try to have one without the others makes us lost. They are all part of our experiencing life fully."[102]

Kiki Athanassoulias of Meal Garden says, "Food and diet are only an element of health, just something in our toolbox. Find what activates your happiness/genius and do more of that. Nourishing your body helps you to be the best you can be." Kiki also says not to look at it as something else to add to the to-do list, but instead to approach it

---

101   Lisa Powell, interview with author on June 29, 2017.

102   Pedram Shojai, OMD, interview with author on July 7, 2017.

with excitement, joy, and gratitude because most of us have so much nutritious food and herbs right at our fingertips. "Look at it as a way of upgrading your choices to get where you want to be."[103]

Josh Gitalis, CN, IFMCP, is a believer in "the fundamentals of health." He says that without all of them, nothing works! They are sleep, movement, healthy food, stress-processing activities, clean water, and a life passion! He admits that habits can be hard to form and reminds us of how it works in the brain. When you start something new, you're literally changing connections in the nervous system. It's like learning to walk—your motor skills improve by making more neural connections in the brain. He compares it to how paths are made in the forest. The path was once thick brush, but by being walked on over and over again, the brush was eventually cleared and a path was made. What's the lesson here? Don't be surprised at the difficulty of starting lifestyle changes. Just imagine that you're literally working to create new highways in your brain! It may be hard work, but the payoff is well worth it when you don't have to depend on medication or fall victim to your circumstances but instead have a new body and mind that works the way it was meant to, confident and happier than ever! Josh likes to refer to the payoff of healthy habits as "health compounding interest." He suggests you start building on one thing (just one!) then continue adding new behaviors onto the first habit. One donut a day usually leads to many other bad behaviors, the results of which can't end well. On the other hand, one apple a day usually leads to many other good behaviors, the results of which *will* end much better. I like Josh's advice: "The best way to get started is to get started!" Don't overthink it. Just do it!

---

103   Kiki Athanassoulias, interview with author on July 28, 2017.

Josh says our biggest threat is chronic degenerative diseases, but they don't happen overnight. It happens after many years of neglecting one's health, while the vitality of the cells slowly wastes away. Each cell in your body has four to seven times the capacity of what's needed to function, which makes your body very resilient, but not forever. He says the current statistics show that one in every two people will have cancer in their lifetime! Our health is only getting worse, and our health care system is clearly strained and overwhelmed.[104] Is that what you're depending on to save you, or are you planning an independent, free future for yourself and your family? Our futures are made by every choice we make *today*!

> *"Small, Smart Choices + Consistency +*
> *Time = RADICAL DIFFERENCE."*[105]
>
> —Darren Hardy

Your Story

What if you were diagnosed with a life-threatening disease and only had a limited amount of time to live? Maybe you're already in that position. How would you answer the following questions? There's just one more key detail: It's a diagnosis that *you* can control...

Would your food choices be different?

How would your relationships be different?

Would you give as much time to mindless TV, FB, and magazines?

---

104 Josh Gitalis, interview with author on September 8, 2017.
105 Hardy, 10.

How would your conversations change? Would you gossip as much?

Would you keep the same relationships?

What contributions would you make?

Could you leave your mark on the world?

How would you spend your time differently?

Where would you go?

What messages would you feed your mind?

Would you find more ways to enjoy life?

How would your thoughts be different?

Would you take the pill, chemo, radiation, or surgery, or would you consider alternative choices?

Would your spirituality deepen?

Would you make your dreams a reality after all?

Would your idea of success change?

Would you see things differently?

Would you learn something new or teach others?

What are you waiting for? You don't need a diagnosis. It could be too late! Are you looking for a cure or for healing? Bill Di Stanisloa of Farm Life Foundation says, "Too many people are looking for a quick fix instead of allowing themselves the time and work to heal." Are you ready to pay now or pay later? I really prefer to say you'll be paying double when you pay later, as problems often get so complex they're costlier than the money and effort it takes to prevent them from happening in the first place. Bill suggests you "take the opportunity now to feel the fear of death. At that moment you can choose to live, allowing you to surrender to the opportunity of change. You don't have to wait for the stimulus of a diagnosis because you can make change this moment. When you *decide*, change begins."[106]

---

106 Bill Di Stanisloa, interview with author on June 27, 2017.

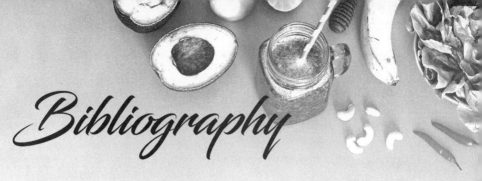

Bibliography

Alexander, Kristy. Interview with author on July 6, 2017.

Allison, Nan, MS, RD, and Carol Beck, MS. *Full & Fulfilled: The Science of Eating to Your Soul's Satisfaction.* Nashville: AB Books, 1998, 2000.

Athanassoulias, Kiki. Interview with author on July 28, 2017.

Bailor, Jonathan. *The Calorie Myth: How to Eat More, Exercise Less, Lose Weight, and Live Better.* New York: HarperCollins Publishers, 2014.

Campbell, T. Colin, PhD, and Thomas M. Campbell II, MD. *The China Study: Startling Implications for Diet, Weight Loss, and Long-Term Health.* Dallas: BenBella Books Inc., 2006.

Calton, Mira and Jayson. *Naked Calories: Discover How Micronutrients Can Maximize Weight Loss, Prevent Disease and Enhance Your Life.* Howard Beach: Changing Lives Press, 2012.

Christianson, Alan, NMD. *The Adrenal Reset Diet: Strategically Cycle Carbs and Proteins to Lose Weight, Balance Hormones, and Move from Stressed to Thriving.* New York: Harmony Books, 2014.

David, Marc. *Nourishing Wisdom: A Mind-Body Approach to Nutrition and Well-Being.* New York: Bell Tower, 1991.

Davis, William, MD. *Wheat Belly: Lose the Wheat, Lose the Weight, and Find Your Path Back to Health.* New York: Rodale, 2011.

Di Stanisloa, Bill. Interview with author on June 27, 2017.

Duke, Dr. Ellan. Interview with author on June 22, 2017.

Ferguson, Greg. Interview with author on June 29, 2017.

Gitalis, Josh. Interview with author on September 8, 2017.

Gottfried, Sara, MD. *The Hormone Cure: Reclaim Balance, Sleep, and Sex Drive; Lose Weight; Feel Focused, Vital, and Energized Naturally with the Gottfried Protocol.* New York: Scribner, 2014.

Hyman, Mark, MD. *The UltraMind Solution: The Simple Way to Defeat Depression, Overcome Anxiety, and Sharpen Your Mind.* New York: Scribner, 2007.

Hardy, Darren. *The Compound Effect: Jumpstart Your Income, Your Life, Your Success.* New York: Vanguard Press, 2010.

Hekler, E. B., C. D. Garnder, and T. N. Robinson, "Effects of a College Course About Food and Society on Students' Eating Behaviors." *American Journal of Preventative Medicine* 38, no. 5 (May 2010): 543–47.

Jamieson, Alexandra. *Women, Food, and Desire: Honor Your Cravings, Embrace Your Desires, Reclaim Your Body.* New York: Gallery Books, 2015.

Kelly, Justine. Interview with author on June 29, 2017.

Keslar, Amie. Interview with author on June 23, 2017.

Lehrer, Jonah. *How We Decide.* New York: First Mariner Books, 2009.

Levine, H., N. Jørgensen, A. Martino-Andrade, J. Mendiola, D. Weksler-Derri, I. Mindlis, R. Pinotti, and S. H. Swan, "Temporal Trends in Sperm Count: A Systematic Review and Meta-Regression Analysis." *Hum Reprod Update* 1;23(6) (Nov 2017):646–659.

Levitt, Andy. Interview with author on July 18, 2017.

Living Planet Index, http://www.livingplanetindex.org/home/index (accessed January 26, 2018).

Lizotte, Jonathan. Interview with author on June 21, 2017.

Manning, Brennan. *Abba's Child: The Cry of the Heart for Intimate Belonging.* Colorado Springs: NavPress, 1994.

Minger, Denise. *Death by Food Pyramid: How Shoddy Science, Sketchy Politics and Shady Special Interests Ruined Your Health... and How to Reclaim It!.* Malibu: Primal Blueprint Publishing, 2013.

Morris, Z. S., S. Wooding S., and Grant J. "The Answer Is 17 years, What Is the Question: Understanding Time Lags in Translational Research." *J R Soc Med* 104, 12 (Dec 2011):510–20.

Moss, Michael. *Salt Sugar Fat: How the Food Giants Hooked Us*. New York: Random House, 2013.

Neill, Michael. *Supercoach: 10 Secrets to Transform Anyone's Life.* New York: Hay House Inc., 2009.

Nymag.com, www.nymag.com/scienceofus/2016/05/you-will-make-200-decisions-about-food-today.html (accessed January 22, 2018).

O'Bryan, Tom, DC, CCN, DACBN. *The Autoimmune Fix: How to Stop the Hidden Autoimmune Damage That Keeps You Sick, Fat, and Tired Before It Turns into Disease.* New York: Rodale, 2016.

Perlmutter, David, MD with Loberg, Kristin. *Grain Brain: The Surprising Truth About Wheat, Carbs, and Sugar – Your Brain's Silent Killers.* New York: Hachette Book Group, 2013.

Pollan, Michael. *The Omnivore's Dilemma: A Natural History of Four Meals.* New York: Penguin Group, 2006.

Powell, Lisa. Interview with author on June 29, 2017.

Rose, Darya, PhD. *Foodist: Using Real Food and Real Science to Lose Weight without Dieting.* New York: Harper One, 2013.

Rosenthal, Joshua. *Integrative Nutrition: Feed Your Hunger for Health & Happiness.* New York: Integrative Nutrition Publishing, 2008.

Rountree, Dr. Robert. Interview with author on July 14, 2017.

Rozman, Deborah and Childre, Doc. *Stopping Emotional Eating: Heartmath Stress and Weight Management Program.* Cardiff: Waterfront Digital Press, 2017.

Rozman, Deborah. Interview with author on July 13, 2017.

Ruiz, Don Miguel. *The Four Agreements: A Practical Guide to Personal Freedom.* San Rafael: Amber-Allen Publishing, 1997.

Shojai, Pedram, OMD. *The Art of Stopping Time: Practical Mindfulness for Busy People.* New York: Rodale, 2017.

Stollmeyer, Rick. Interview with author on July 21, 2017.

Terkeurst, Lysa. *Made to Crave: Satisfying Your Deepest Desire with God, Not Food.* Grand Rapids: Zondervan, 2010.

Telpner, Meghan. *UnDiet: The Shiny, Happy, Vibrant, Gluten-Free, Plant-Based Way to Look Better, Feel Better, and Live Better Each and Every Day!*. Guilford: Skirt!, 2013.

TheDr.com. www.thedr.com/all-about-gluten/articles/intestinal-problems-and-wthole-body-symptoms-gut-101-the-effect-of-foods-as-written-for-autism-one (accessed January 22, 2018).

Thomsen, Dori. Interview with author on June 26, 2017.

Warner, Melanie. *Pandora's Lunchbox: How Processed Food Took Over the American Meal*. New York: Scribner. 2013

Wolf, Robb. *Wired to Eat: Turn Off Cravings, Rewire Your Appetite for Weight Loss, and Determine the Foods That Work for You*. New York: Harmony Books, 2017.

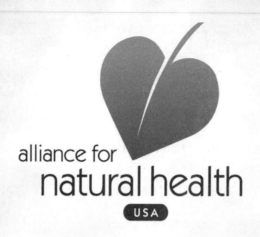

alliance for
natural health
USA

The Alliance for Natural Health USA (ANH-USA) is a national non-profit dedicated to shifting the conventional medical paradigm from an exclusive focus on surgery, drugs, and treating the symptoms of disease to a proactive and preventive approach focusing on a nutrient-rich diet, proper supplementation, and limiting exposure to toxic substances. We mobilize an army of over 500,000 members to defend consumer access to safe dietary supplements, uphold meaningful organic standards, and fight monopolistic practices that threaten integrative and alternative health practitioners. We also protect access to vital individualized compounded medications, call out government collusion with Big Pharma and Big Food, and defend people's right to vaccine choice.

Join the Fight:

www.ANH-USA.org

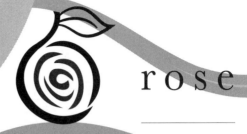

apple rose

Apple Rose Beauty provides you with luxurious, natural and organic face care and beauty products that work to visibly alleviate tough skin issues such as oily skin, dry skin, acne, acne scars and signs of aging. Our unique formulations are crafted with the most potent, pure and premium natural, wildcrafted and certified organic ingredients sourced from around the globe. Named after two victims of human trafficking, our company has a big heart with a mission to employ human trafficking survivors and support organizations involved in their rescue and rehabilitation.

https://tinyurl.com/
AppleRoseBeauty

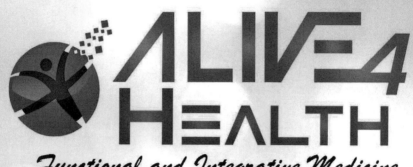

ALIVE4 HEALTH

Functional and Integrative Medicine

Alive4Health is located at:
410 Jacksonville Drive, Jacksonville Beach,
FL 32250 +1 904 712 3737

Dr. Ellan Duke * Dr. Marty Monahan * Dr. Linda Quinn

At Alive4Health, our team of healthcare providers passionately seeks to facilitate Whole Health (mind, body and spirit) with cutting-edge, safe and efficient solutions for health challenges and optimal performance.

Your care here begins with a full body computerized diagnostic evaluation with our AO Scan. This technology is known as Bioenergetic Testing with Radionics and produces a 24-page health report. It is 85–95% accurate compared to other available medical testing. This comprehensive program is utilized for disease prevention and early detection. It may indicate the presence of bacteria, viruses, parasites, mold, fungus, heavy metal toxicity, trace mineral deficits, hormone imbalance and amino acid profile as well as food and airborne allergies.

From here we are able to create solution steps for improving many health concerns and returning your body to its peak function. Personalized and specific protocols may include IV Nutrition, Frequency Therapies, Hyperbaric Oxygen, K Laser, Acoustic Light Wave, Acupuncture, Genetic Testing, Hormone Replacement Therapy and Stem Cell Therapy.

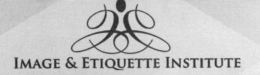

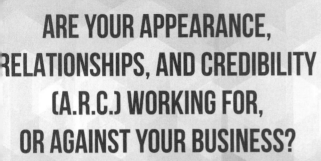
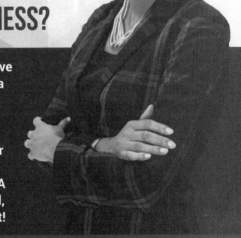

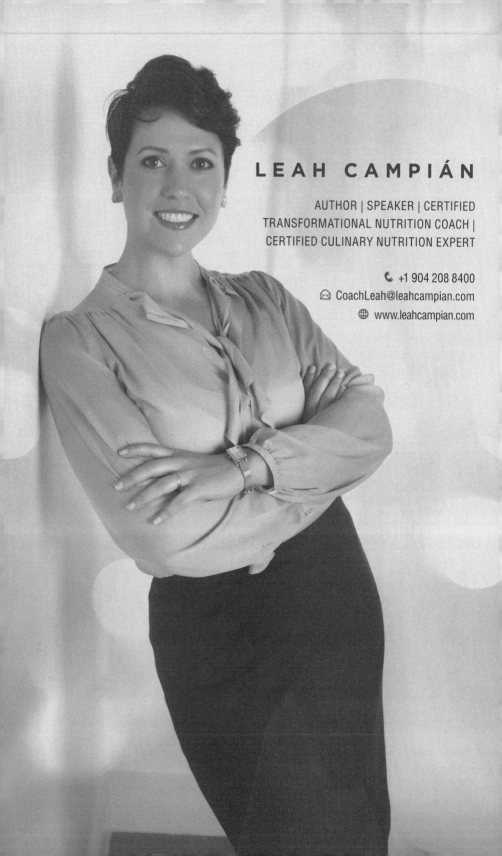

LEAH CAMPIÁN

AUTHOR | SPEAKER | CERTIFIED
TRANSFORMATIONAL NUTRITION COACH |
CERTIFIED CULINARY NUTRITION EXPERT

📞 +1 904 208 8400
✉ CoachLeah@leahcampian.com
🌐 www.leahcampian.com

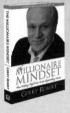
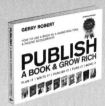
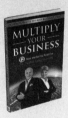
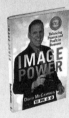
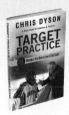
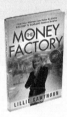
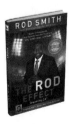
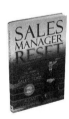

OTHER BOOKS RECOMMENDED BY BLACK CARD BOOKS

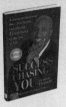

Success Chasing You
A Journey to Discovering
One's True Purpose and
Achieving Greatness
in Any Area of Life
Travon Taylor
ISBN: 978-1-77204-841-4

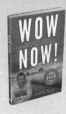

WOW Now!
The NEW Guide To
Reclaim An Abundant
And Spectacular Life
Florin Pasat
ISBN: 978-1-77204-300-6

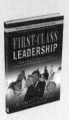

First-Class Leadership
How Highly Effective
Teams Can Achieve
Breakthrough Results
Hamid Safaei
ISBN: 978-1-77204-760-8

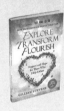

Explore, Transform, Flourish
Support and Hope for
Those Who Help Others
How Professionals
Keep It Together
Gillian Stevens
ISBN: 978-1-77204-837-7

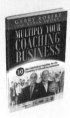

Multiply Your Coaching Business
10 New Marketing
Realities for the Coaching
& Consulting Industries
Gerry Robert and
Kevin Judge, CEC
ISBN: 978-1-77371-050-1

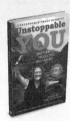

Unstoppable You
Exceed Uncertainties,
Embrace Possibilities,
Earn Independence
Unstoppable Tracy Schmitt
ISBN: 978-1-77204-915-2

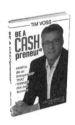

Be a CASHpreneur®
How to Be an Entrepreneur
THAT THRIVES
Not Just Survives
Tim Voss
ISBN: 978-1-77204-963-3

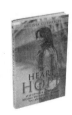

The Heart Of Hope
Step Up Your Game And
Become The Strong Woman
You KNOW You Are!
Melissa Cuturich
ISBN: 978-1-77204-573-4

POWERED BY

www.blackcardbooks.com